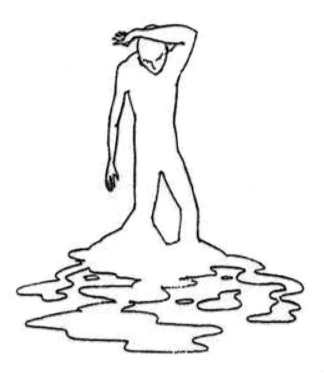

Information contained in this book should not be used to alter a medically prescribed regimen or as a form of self treatment. Consult a licensed physician before beginning this or any other exercise program.

2nd Edition Copywrite © 2004

3rd Edition Copywrite © 2010

LMA Publishing and Dr. Jane Pentz

Cover illustration by Emmett Aeillo

Printed in the United States of America

ISBN 978-1-892426-16-1

LMA Publishing

www.lifestylemanagement.com

email:info@lifestylemanagement.com

fax: 800.617.4615

# Nutrition Specialists

Visit www.aasdn.org for a list of qualified personal trainers who are also Nutrition Specialists. They can work with you to provide you with a total fitness program.

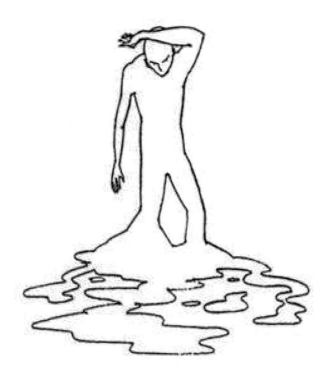

# Take Charge of Your Health - Today!

# Contents

# This Book Belongs To:

Name _____

Street Address _____

City _____ State _____ Zip _____

Phone _____

E-mail _____

Welcome to the beginning of a new life;  a life in which you are in charge - no one else - of your health.  No more excuses.  Yes, you have no control over what life may throw at you.  But there is much you do have control over.  So today is the first day of taking control.

Remember,  it is "selfish" not to make your health your top priority. After all, if your body breaks down you can't be that great son or daughter, that great mom or dad, that great husband or wife, that great athlete or scholar, that great brother or sister, .........

So stay brave and don't let anything get in your way.

# Dr. Jane's Story

I often question this passion that drives me in my work. Why do I get angry when I read about another labeling lie, or another false claim concerning some new product that will "cure" all that ails us? Why do I feel compelled to convince people that they must stop making excuses and take charge of their health? Understanding my past is critical to understanding this passion.

A good portion of my life was spent on surviving psychologically. My daily energy was spent on *coping*. If you have been there, or are there now, you know exactly what I am talking about. My day was spent trying to make life perfect around me so that I wouldn't be screamed at or ridiculed. I had no self-esteem or self-confidence. Happiness was something that occurred in fleeting moments. I can best describe those fleeting moments as "absence of emotional pain". I had spent my life living a lie and being a fake. I had convinced myself that I was stupid, a lousy mother and a lousy wife.

I had a very emotional incident that occurred over 15 years ago which changed my life. That incident, convinced me, beyond doubt, that I was special, that I possessed talents and qualities that made me unique. My goal at the time was to find peace. I had no idea what form that peace would take. I only knew that I could no longer be what everyone wanted me to be - I had to be myself. But first, I had to figure out just who I was. Who lived inside this body? I not only had to find out who I was, but then I had to accept who I was.

The whole process was terrifying.  Peace came when I realized no matter who lived inside my body, that person would be a fundamentally good person - dysfunctional yes - but good. I found my family and friends still loved me. As a matter of fact, they loved me even more.

My life began to change dramatically. At that time my oldest daughter was having difficulties adjusting to school. My precious  sweet little girl was being perceived by teachers as a trouble maker. She was everything but. How could she be labeled as a defiant child in kindergarten?

For the first time in my life I took charge of the problem and began to search for solutions. My baby girl was having problems concentrating. She was diagnosed as "hyperactive". I began to read everything I could get my hands on about hyperactivity in children. It soon became apparent that many of her problems were aggravated by certain foods; i.e. sugars and chemicals.  It was then that I decided to go back to school to learn everything I could about foods and allergies.

I was terrified. I had been a poor student in high school (to put it mildly). A high school teacher (dear Mr. Walsh)  had convinced me that I was much too stupid to  go to college. But my motivational levels were great; I was going to help my daughter.

To my amazement, after completing some remedial work at a community college, I discovered I wasn't stupid - I actually did very well. A very dear and special friend, Dr. Pat Poggi, supported, encouraged, and convinced me to apply for acceptance into a nutrition program at Vassar College. Not only was I accepted, but I completed the nutritional biochemistry program, and graduated with honors. How could this stupid girl actually graduate from Vassar? Anything is possible!

While at Vassar, I met my mentor, Dr. Marcie Greenwood. She convinced me that I had been bright all along and she provided the emotional support I needed to continue my education.

With Dr. Greenwood's help, I applied to graduate school. I was accepted into a combined masters and Ph.D. program at Tufts University. My graduate program consisted of completing fitness evaluations and nutritional analyses on 250 women over 60. I completed the 4 year program in 5 years (I was told we older people take a little longer).

I also met my husband while at Tufts and learned that the peace I had found was only the beginning. Beyond peace came a great happiness. I found someone very special to share "Jane" with.

Upon graduation, I once again experienced a feeling of being lost. What was I going to do now? After several months, and almost by accident, I fell into the world of fitness and continuing education. I slowly developed the Nutrition Specialist Course, an 18 hour nutrition certification course for professionals. With the help of wonderful friends, and inspirational students, the course was presented to a national audience in 1997. I finally realized what I wanted to do when I grew up (or rather grew older).

Today my students still use the word "passionate" to describe my teaching. Upon examining this passion, I realize it was always there. I just had to unleash it.

I am convinced that we are all unique individuals. We are all a "one of a kind". If I can do it, everyone can. I am no more unique or special than anyone else; but unique and special we are. I am also convinced that to search our souls, find that uniqueness, and live the passion within, is fundamental to happiness. The loss of **one**, non-developed, non discovered, unique individual is a loss to **all** the world.

I implore you to discover your passion, and share your "greatness" with the world. And just as importantly, I implore you to take care of your body so that you can have a place to live while discovering, developing, and sharing this passion - your uniqueness - with the world. You can do it! Slow, small steps is all it takes.

# Introduction

As a doctor of nutrition, I have worked in the field of fitness for almost a decade. I have worked with and lectured to thousands of people. By far, the most difficult part of my job has been convincing people to make healthy living their top priority.

For years I have been searching for that special phrase or that all inclusive picture that would convey the critical nature of placing individual health above all other priorities, i.e. that picture that would be worth a thousand words. I want to thank my colleague and friend, Robert Montague for that phrase and the title of this book, *If You Don't Take Care Of Your Body Where Are You Going To Live*. The moment I heard it I knew that this was the phrase I had been searching for. My hope is that the title of this book will convince you of the necessity of taking care of your body and the futility of all other goals in comparison.

This book is dedicated to all of us who get caught up in doing "what is imminent" rather than what is truly important to us. We get so entrenched in our daily activities that we forget to take the time to take care of our bodies - the only one we will have (at least here on this earth).

The goal of this book is to convince you that the quality of your life and your relationship to others depends on the fact that you must have a place to live. We are a replacement society - if the car or TV breaks down, we simply replace it. We cannot replace our bodies. There is no buying another one. Many people believe that a miracle-working physician, or a miracle drug will fix their bodies if they break down. The fact is, degenerative diseases of old age (heart disease, cancer, diabetes, hypertension, etc.) are chronic diseases; they do not go away. They may subside temporarily, but they are incurable. The key to conquering them is to do what we can to prevent them from occurring in the first place.

**The evidence is too great to ignore the facts any longer.** There is a direct relationship between the food we eat, our physical activity level, our stress level and long-term health. Yes, genetics does play a part. Genetics is similar to an analogy comparing our bodies to cars. Some of us are given a compact car to get through life, while others are given a big luxurious limousine. Both will get us through life, but even the limousine will end up in the junk yard if we don't take care of it. Remember, we alone are responsible for our health even through our senior years. We must all leave this world one day, but how and when we do is partially under our control.

Part I (Where Are You Going To Live) of this book deals with stories of the sad life experiences of others. These experiences are an attempt to convince you of the futility of not putting your health first. We can not do it for anyone else, nor can anyone else do it for us.

Part II (A Call to Action) contains stories of other, very busy people, who have struggled, or are still struggling with keeping their priorities in perspective. In Part II (No Excuses) I will ask you to look at the excuses you make that prevent you from putting your health first. I will then guide you through several steps in learning to "take charge of your health".

Part III (The Basics) is the academics of healthy living. This section deals with the components of exercise and eating as they relate to health, not how you will look in spandex. There are no magic pills. Think of exercise, healthy eating, and stress reduction as the tools to maintaining your only home.

Part IV (Menu Planning for a Healthy Lifestyle) is the resource you will need to determine your individual menu plan. Part V (Recipes) contains easy, complete recipes designed to help you get started on your menu planning.

Healthy living doesn't require a lot of time; what it does require is making a commitment to ourselves, and keeping that commitment. Steven Covey, in his book, *The Seven Habits of Highly Effective People,* describes integrity as making and keeping promises to ourselves. Taking care of ourselves takes on a new meaning when it is no longer perceived as selfish, but as a positive character trait. **It is selfish *not* to take charge of our health**.

Finally, my prayer is that this book will convey the importance of putting your health first, and the realization that once you have worked through all of your excuses, the implementation of a healthy lifestyle can actually be easy and fun. The process of change, while seemingly slow, should not and must not be an overwhelming experience.

Of course, there are no guarantees. I cannot promise you longevity or guarantee health. What I can promise you is that you will have more energy, feel better about yourself, and have a brighter outlook on life.

I wish you the *Best of health.*

*Dr. Jane*

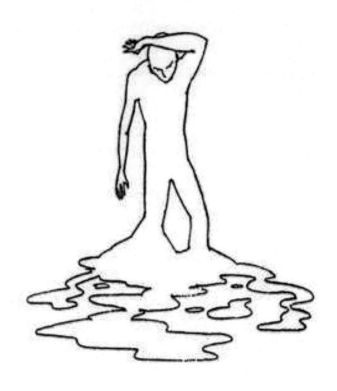

# Part I

# Where Are You Going to Live?

# Where Are You Going To Live?

I'm sure most of us as we look back on our lives and experiences have all known someone who died prematurely - taken from this life long before old age. Some of these deaths were not preventable. The death of Princess Dianna filled the world with sadness and grief. Here was a charismatic woman who overcame such odds as bulimia, and even national scorn. After years of suffering, she had begun to experience happiness; and then, in an instant, she was pulled from the world - and at such a young age. How unfair!

Five days after the death of Princess Diana, Mother Theresa died at the age of 87. Most of us were equally saddened by her death; yet there was not that same sense of tragedy. After all, Mother Theresa lived a long and productive life. All generations will remember both women, one name will convey tragedy while the other will convey the essence of life - we are born and we die.

This section is not about death, but about life. The statistics indicate that most of us will live to see old age. That's the good news. The bad news is that some of us will acquire one or more forms of a chronic disease, either disabling us or reducing the quality of our lives. The Journal of the American Medical Society indicates that chronic disease is on the rise affecting nearly 100 million Americans in 1995. By the year 2020 this figure is expected to reach 134 million.

Our nation is in jeopardy - chronic diseases are occurring in epidemic proportions. The Surgeon General, in conjunction with The American College of Sports Medicine and the Center for Disease Control have issued a call to action. Many of the chronic diseases affecting Americans can be reduced, and in some cases eliminated.

But Americans are not responding to this call. Why? Americans are among the brightest people in the world. Why are we not making the changes necessary to improve the quality of our lives?

I believe the answer lies in the way we, as Americans, view life. Our top priority is making a living; a necessity to be sure. Without food, shelter, and clothing life becomes painful - pleasure and joy are lost.

Our hectic lifestyles prevent us from taking the time to contemplate what is truly important. We have daytimers under our arms helping us to make the most of every moment. We have email and pagers, all in the name of maximizing efficiency. But there comes a time when we must ask ourselves where in the world are we going? Without direction, we simply continue to run around in circles.

This section is designed to help you stop running long enough to take a look at where you are going. The good news is, we do have control over how *our* story will end!

# Mrs. T's Story

I met Mrs. T over 30 years ago. I actually married into her family. At that time she was in her late twenties, married with two children and a third child on the way. Mrs. T was a very attractive, happy woman who loved to laugh - she laughed loud and often. She made everyone laugh. Anyone who knew Mrs. T knew her for her laugh.

Mr. T was a very large man that didn't laugh very much. He loved to eat, drink, and smoke. He was pleasant enough, but all conversations centered on how "rotten" the world was. He had been a laborer all his life with a large company that paid him very well. He was often argumentative and actually seemed to enjoy picking fights. One thing was sure - Mr. and Mrs. T were in love.

At age 36, Mr. T had a stroke. Although it was serious, he had no long term disabilities. Within a few months he was back to work. His physician told him he had to quit smoking and drinking, begin an exercise program, and eat healthier. He was also instructed to take his medication daily.

For the next several months Mrs. T didn't laugh much. Mr. T followed none of the advice prescribed by his physician. Mrs. T, concerned and worried, began to nag her husband. After several months she stopped nagging. She began to laugh again.

I remember a conversation Mrs. T had with her sister while in my company. Mrs. T's sister was admonishing her; "Why don't you make your husband take his medication and make him quit smoking? He's going to die if you don't".

I will forever remember Mrs. T's response. "I'm not his mother", Mrs. T said. "I tried nagging." "We did nothing but fight and started hating each other." "I realized I can not make him do anything. " "My choices are to get divorced and bury him or stay married to him and bury him."

Bury him she did. Six years later, to the day, Mr. T died at the age of 42 of a massive stroke. He left his lovely wife and three children, ages 8 to 15. Mrs. T didn't laugh for a long time.

Today she is once again laughing. Her children are grown and she has lovely grandchildren. She has never remarried.

**We are all in charge of our own health!**

# Mr. P's Story

Mr. P is in his mid fifties. He has been seriously ill for over 10 years. It's been one health disaster after another. Mr. P smoked since he was thirteen years old. Several years ago he had to have one of his lungs removed. He quit smoking several months before the surgery.

Two years ago Mr. P had his first heart attack. Ironically, he was not over-weight, nor had he even been overweight. After his heart attack, Mr. P was forced by his HMO to enroll in a program designed to help him make lifestyle changes. He began a walking program and a nutritionist designed a healthy eating plan.

Mr. P followed the exercise program for about six months. His family was not very supportive. They made fun of "the old man" walking. His wife refused to make separate meals for him. "It's not a little butter that's the problem", she would say. She would explain to friends about how he had given up smoking, was exercising, was not overweight, and hence, "there was no need to be neurotic about his eating". After about six months Mr. P's motivation began to wane, and one year after his first heart attack he was no longer exercising. He was still skipping breakfast, eating two hot dogs and fries almost every day for lunch, and his wife continued cooking the same meals she always had.

Several weeks ago, Mr. P was rushed to the hospital and had to undergo surgery again because of extensive arterial blockage. This time Mr. P's doctors frightened him. They convinced him that he had to make changes in his lifestyle or he would not live to see old age.

Mr. P has made a promise to himself that he will exercise again, and this time he says he will "stick" to it. His wife has agreed to accompany him to see the nutritionist.

Mr. P's story is not over yet. He has been given another chance. He has decided to take this warning seriously and make the necessary lifestyle changes.

**Stay Tuned!**

# Mrs. Y's Story

Mrs. Y is retired. She is over 65 years old and lives with her husband in a modest retirement home. She worked all her life and enjoys retirement. Her husband has had 2 heart attacks, smokes, is overweight, and does not exercise.

Mrs. Y is also overweight, and has been diagnosed with diabetes. She has kept her appointments with her dietician. She knows she needs to exercise and make changes in her eating patterns. She really tries to follow her "diet", but, as she explains, "there are just so many things that get in the way". "My husband complains if I change the way I cook, and I can't leave him to go exercise".

The excuses abound: "I've tried to cook my own foods, but it's so much work to cook two separate meals"; "I have to bake cookies and cakes for my friends when they come over and I can't stop myself from eating them"; "my friends tell me I'm not really that overweight - several people they know with diabetes are actually a lot "bigger" than I am"; "I would like to walk, but it's too cold outside"; "I go shopping almost every other day and that counts as walking". The excuses go on and on.

Mrs. Y doesn't feel well. She complains to friends that her eyesight is deteriorating fast. She has trouble sleeping. Some nights just lying flat in her bed causes her pain. She has urinary infections that are never ending. But all of these ailments, she says, are due to getting old, not the diabetes.

Mrs. Y has one very kind special friend that gently advises her to talk to her doctor about all of these ailments. She asks Mrs. Y to walk with her, even when it is cold outside. She also shares her heart healthy recipes with Mrs. Y, hoping that she will begin to cook better for herself and her husband. This lovely friend has none of the ailments that Mrs. Y has and loves Mrs. Y like a sister. She also knows that she can't make Mrs. Y take care of herself. For Christmas, this friend gave Mrs. Y a book, "*Make the Connection*" written by Oprah Winfrey. Mrs. Y promises she will read it. Maybe she will and maybe she will begin to take care of herself. Maybe not.

**Stay Tuned!**

# Mr. G's Story

Mr. G came to see me after his third heart attack. He was not sitting in front of me because he wanted to; he was sitting in front of me because his wife had made the appointment.

After his first heart attack, Mr. G's physician told him to quit smoking, change his eating patterns, and begin an exercise program. He did none of the above. After his second heart attack, Mr. G gave up smoking. I asked him what convinced him to quit smoking. "While I was in intensive care", he replied, "I learned that twenty-nine out of the thirty people in the cardiac intensive care unit were smokers". "So that scared you", I asked? "No", he commented. "It just made me realize how great a risk factor smoking is; so I gave it up". "My wife thinks she nagged me into it; but I gave it up because I wanted to".

After our second consultation, it was clear that Mr. G had no intention of exercising or changing his eating patterns. I remember asking him if there was anything I could say to convince him to begin a walking program, or to begin eating a healthy breakfast. I still remember the honest look on his face as he answered with an emphatic "NO". "Why", I asked!! "Don't you want to be around to see your grandchildren grow up?" "Sure, but not enough to start a stupid exercise program or eat the same foods my wife tries to make me eat", he replied. "I like my butter and Scotch."

I suggested small changes; perhaps a ten minute walk per day and maybe a Scotch every other day. Mr. G simply laughed. I was amazed! "Aren't these small changes easier and less painful than going through surgery again", I asked. He laughed again and answered, "You sound like my wife".

There was nothing I could to say to convince Mr. G to change his lifestyle. I suggested counseling, but he once again laughed.

Mr. G had his fourth heart attack 6 months ago, and this one killed him. He will never see his grandchildren grow up.

**We cannot do it for anyone else, no matter how much we love them.**

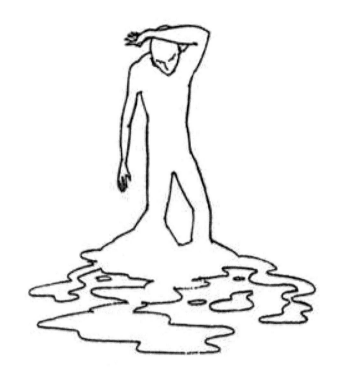

# Part II
# A Call to Action

# A Call to Action

The state of our Nation is in jeopardy - we are in the grips of an epidemic which is now the # 2 killer of Americans. This epidemic isn't viral, but is associated with the American lifestyle - this epidemic is <u>obesity.</u> The Surgeon General has issued a call to action.

The purpose of this section is to convince you of the necessity to heed this call to action personally. You can begin to make small lifestyle changes that will make huge differences in your health and ultimately in the health of our nation.

The following are stories about people who, despite their hectic lives or limited physical abilities, have made the decision to take charge of their health.

# Sarah's Story

Sarah may appear to be like any other small business owner; she runs a service for busy dog owners, walking dogs four times a day for 40 minutes at a time. In October, 1995 anybody who knew Sarah would find it inconceivable that she could handle the physical exertion of walking. It would have been a daunting, if not impossible, task.

Sarah was diagnosed with Lupus in 1990. By October, 1995 she suffered from Lupus, epilepsy and arthritis. Her deteriorating joints ached, and she wore cumbersome braces which stretched from her hips to mid-calves and was about to be custom-fitted for her next set. She could do very little without becoming fatigued.

Sarah had been through physical therapy off and on for a period of five years, often going three times per week. It did help, but she never regained much muscle strength, and the effects were short-lived. While seeking relief through physical therapy Sarah also sought help from diet programs. Many of the programs promised fantastic results within unrealistic time frames and failed to deliver, and she didn't learn much about nutrition.

Sarah was on 20 different medications, and while she respected her doctors, she had reached the point where she knew she needed to make a change. "I was frustrated and ready for something to change my life", she said, thinking back to that October, "and ready to make the commitment".

That's when Sarah phoned me. We had first met at a meeting of the South Shore Lupus chapter. It was a call that Sarah claims changed her way of life.

During Sarah's first meeting with me we discussed her goals and I informed her it would take approximately two years to reach her ideal body fat. By August, 1996, just ten months later, Sarah had only six percent more to lose in order to reach her goal. In addition, she had experienced fewer flare-ups for shorter periods of time, didn't wear braces, was able to discontinue some of her medication and was experiencing little joint pain.

The road to better health, however, was strewn with obstacles and setbacks. After a few weeks of altering her eating habits and exercising with weights, Sarah began to notice positive changes; she lost inches and her body composition improved. But six weeks into her program she experienced a serious setback when her Lupus flared. She had no appetite and couldn't keep much of what she ate down, which forced her to stop exercising. For three weeks in November, 1995 Sarah was frustrated; she had to start "back at zero". When she began her program again, she had to proceed slowly, and she couldn't do as many repetitions of her exercises. Her health problems of epilepsy, Lupus, and arthritis slowed her down; it took longer compared to other people that started when she did.

19

Sarah once again began to see benefits; strengthening exercises improved her muscle strength and eliminated joint pain. She was encouraged to keep working by the extra support, encouragement and motivation she received from her trainer and her doctors. Sarah did experience another bout in mid-January and one in February, but they were not as severe and lasted for shorter periods of time. As of August 1996, she has not experienced another flare-up and considers herself to be "in remission".

Sarah's achievements surpassed all her expectations. She continues to see me for periodic checkups. The only pills she takes now are a multi vitamin and a vitamin E tablet. When asked about her present condition Sarah says, "I'm leading more of a normal life than I have in the last six years since I was diagnosed with Lupus." She has more energy and mobility, her muscles are stronger and she no longer misses foods and substances she's given up, such as caffeine that attenuated her seizures.

Sarah is both realistic and optimistic about her future. "There is no cure for Lupus, but for now I can enjoy how good I feel, how healthy I feel and the money I save on medication. I hope it stays in remission....". "Right now I'm enjoying the freedom". Looking back on her experience Sarah says, "I know I found the courage and did the work. My trainer, Dr. Jane, and my other doctors gave me the support and education I needed to get me through it. I now view exercise and healthy eating as my ticket to life".

# Elaine's Story

Elaine is the former fitness director for Lifestyle Management Associates. She taught individuals how to be active, no matter how hectic their lifestyle.

Here is Elaine's story in her own words.

Today at 49 years old I am in the best physical condition of my life, and I am very proud of that fact. By the time my mother was my age she had already experienced near death at childbirth, high blood pressure, high cholesterol, cancer and diabetes. Having witnessed my mother's struggle to live, I vowed that I would do whatever I could do to avoid the physical adversities she faced.

Of course this reality did not hit me until I was in my early twenties, and I was a real chunky short woman. In fact at twenty-three I weighed more than I did at thirty years old and nine months pregnant with my third child. At four feet ten inches tall I was approaching that stage where I was almost as wide as I was tall.

Fortunately, before I got totally out of control I started jogging. Luckily my new husband joined me and together we got ourselves into an active lifestyle. After twenty-seven years of marriage we are still jogging together.

It's difficult to pinpoint when I became an inactive person. I was an active child. Because of my small stature, I was always running to keep up with everyone else, especially my older brother. Even as a teenager I did a lot of walking and I attempted some high school sports. I was definitely not an athlete, but I did like to be active.

I guess I discovered the *love* of exercise after college. I was a Physical Education major in college and was exposed to all forms of athletics. I have to admit that for most sports skills classes I really struggled - I still have nightmares about my swimming and diving course! But it was also at this time that I was exposed to numerous forms of dance and rhythmic gymnastics which I adored.

When I got my first teaching job I was afraid to teach some sports so I focused on movement education. I was able to see the love of movement through my students, and it made me realize that the act of moving my body through space was a joy.

I think that loving what you do is the real key to being an active person for a lifetime. I remembered how much I loved to run, and now I run with a smile on my face. Rollerblading and skiing are also favorite activities, along with dancing whenever I get the chance. Being active makes me feel like a kid again and that is a wonderful feeling at almost 50.

# Don's Story

Don is a very handsome, very fit man in his late 30's. He is an extremely stressed salesperson for a very large corporation. His annual sales are well over $50 million.

Don lives the fast life. He travels constantly and must wine and dine his clients. He is out to sporting events, sales meetings, or dinner meetings almost every evening.

So how does Don stay fit? When traveling, he always stays at hotels that have workout facilities. That's the easy part. The hard part is making the time to exercise.

I asked Don how he makes the time to exercise faithfully. His answer was unexpected. He explained to me that every week he outlines all his meetings, etc., as well as his exercise times. He never writes "exercise" in his computerized daytimer for fear that someone will see it. He disguises these times with codes, such as lunch, traveling, or meeting with "so and so". I asked why he felt compelled to disguise his exercise times. He patiently explained that he didn't want anyone to know he was exercising because it would be perceived as selfish; "there is always so much work to be done that the powers to be would be *upset* if they knew I was taking time to exercise".

My nature forced me to ask Don why he felt he had to lie. "Wouldn't it be easier to be honest and set a great example for other sales personnel (also under extreme stress)?", I asked. Don smiled and again patiently explained that the corporate world wasn't into fitness. He assured me that it would be a huge blow to his career if management discovered he was putting time aside to exercise.

I took his word for it! I certainly didn't want to interfere with his career. As Don's nutritionist, I wasn't concerned with the how; all I knew was he was committed to exercise, and from my perspective, that was the important part.

By far, Don's biggest challenge was learning to eat healthier when traveling, and when dining with clients (which was most of the time). Don has made tremendous lifestyle changes in this area as well. He couches his heathier choices and minimizes his alcohol intake under the guise of having an "ulcer". Again, as Don's nutritionist I am thrilled that he has made these wonderful lifestyle changes.

Don is now working on ways to reduce his stress. He is a great example of how anyone can make healthy lifestyle choices no matter how hectic or stressful the lifestyle.

**Congratulations Don!**

# Karen's Story

I met Karen two years ago when she took my Nutrition Specialist Course. I was impressed with her honest and enthusiastic nature. As the weekend progressed, it was obvious that the entire class was impressed with her candor, and inspirational nature. We were all moved to tears when she shared her touching, life-changing story.

Here is Karen's story in her own words.

Ever since I can remember, I have struggled with my weight and body image. As a result, low self-esteem held me back from following my "heart's dreams.

I put an end to the yo-yo dieting and maintained an exercise program along with a healthy eating plan. My confidence grew and I became certified as an aerobics instructor.

In the years to follow, I continued to maintain what I thought was a healthy and happy lifestyle. I worked as a successful sales representative, taught 7 aerobic classes a week, and gave birth to two beautiful children. Shortly after my son was born, I revisited my internist for what I anticipated to be my best physical exam in years. Within five minutes of the appointment my doctor found a lump on my throat. Shortly after, I was diagnosed with thyroid cancer.

I was terrified. But I slowly began facing my fears and I have since successfully overcome the challenges of cancer. I began to view life very differently. But there was something missing. I started searching, always asking myself, why me? What am I suppose to be learning? What is my purpose in life?

I was determined to find the answers. I started on a new path to find the missing "connection". I had to listen to my heart and expand upon the passion within me. I knew I had to learn more about my body's physical well-being. I became certified in personal training and I became certified as a Nutrition Specialist through Dr. Jane's certification course.

Then I had a "vision"! Yes, a vision. I could see a room, a four seasons sun room where people could come for private training in a motivating, but non-intimidating atmosphere. I knew this room would become a reality someday. This was going to be *the* place where people would come and make the "connection". The room became a reality.

But, I was still searching for some missing pieces to the puzzle. I began to learn a tremendous amount on healing and spirituality. I enrolled in a journal writing class and found a renewed inner strength. Then, knowing very little about yoga, I enrolled in an instructor training program and suddenly the pieces of the puzzle started coming together. I was finally beginning to understand that all roads were leading me to integrate my mind, body, and spirit.

I am working with clients now in my "warm, intimate, inspirational room; and I have discovered that my passion within is what led me to finally making the "connection". I can now work with clients to help them make the connection of mind, body, and spirit - to become whole.

# Mom's Story

The person who most exemplifies the phrase "I'm not getting older - I'm getting better" is my own mother. At 80 years old, she is healthier than many 40 year olds with no ailments.

She turned 80 years old seven days after my dad died. My parents had been married over 60 years, and although Mom sometimes finds the evenings long and lonely, she still loves life. Her positive attitude can certainly be attributed to her good health.

She walks just as fast as I do and can lift my 40 pound granddaughter (her great-granddaughter) over her head. She makes healthy meals for herself every day. She enjoys cooking, reading labels, counting protein grams and servings of fruits and veggies.

She has always been active. She describes how much better she feels when she exercises. She use to walk the high school track near her home. She would walk several miles while encouraging my ailing dad to walk at least once around the track. Last year she joined a small hospital affiliated exercise facility. She learned how to take her heart rate, how to use a treadmill, bike, and rowing machine.

Mom cleans her own home daily and walks to do her laundry at a common laundry room. Most of all, she loves to shop. There have been many times that we shopped until "I dropped". She walks several miles almost everyday just shopping. She also loves her grandchildren and great-grandchildren (she has over 40 great-grandchildren).

My mom is by far the bravest, kindest, and most alive, most vibrant woman I know. She is my heroine and my mentor. I want to be exactly like her when I grow up—or rather grow older.

# No Excuses

Now that you have heard how other people have taken charge of their health, it's time to evaluate your life. Are you still in the blaming stages? Is it someone else's fault that you are overworked, overweight, or unfit? If so, then your first step must be to take responsibility for your own health.

In each of the previous stories, every person learned to take responsibility, no matter what the circumstances, for their health. In some cases there were inspirational individuals that helped the person to change, but in the end no one can force another to change. Each of us must take personal responsibility.

**Responsibility**. Steven Covey in his book, *The Seven Habits of Highly Effective People* defines the word responsibility as the ability to choose our responses. All effective people are what he calls proactive. Proactive people take charge and act, versus reactive people that allow themselves to be acted upon. In essence this means that as human beings we can choose to take responsibility for our own lives.

"Our behavior is a function of our decisions, not our conditions." We all have the ability to choose our responses. We can become responsible, i.e. response-able. Responsible people do not blame circumstances, conditions, or conditioning for their behavior. Persons in the blaming stages are reactive and cannot be successful in long term health and weight management. It will always be something or someone else's fault. This can be a very difficult concept to accept emotionally, especially for people who have experienced years of misery in the name of circumstances. But each of us must come to grips with ourselves and be able to deeply and honestly say "I am what I am today because of the decisions I made yesterday".

This personal response-ability is not about time management. The underlying problem is "self-management". The biggest decision, and it is a decision, is to decide to take control of our lives and ultimately our health. We must each individually open our own "gate" (Covey).

At this point, if you are still in the blaming stages (its your boss's fault, or your spouse's fault, or your childrens' fault, etc.) I suggest you *study Steven Covey's book before continuing*. And I do mean "study". You will never be successful in long term health if you remain in the blaming stages. Only those of you who are ready to take charge of your lives and your health should read on!

## So Are You Ready?

Welcome and congratulations. I guarantee you that you have just completed the most difficult part of your journey to taking charge of your health. I promise you from this point on the journey gets easier, and for many will even be fun.

# Step 1: Proactive

Are you reactive or proactive? Proactive people can be differentiated from reactive people by looking at the language they use:

| REACTIVE LANGUAGE | PROACTIVE LANGUAGE |
|---|---|
| There's nothing I can do. | Let's look at our alternatives. |
| That's just the way I am. | I can choose a different approach. |
| He makes me so mad. | I control my own feelings. |
| I have to do that. | I can create an effective alternative. |
| I must. | I choose. |
| I can't. | I prefer. |
| If only. | I will. |

Becoming proactive requires listening to your internal voice, i.e., examining the scripted language from the accumulation of your past experiences. Take the time now to examine this language. Begin to recognize your reactive phrases. How often do you use these reactive phrases. You can distinguish reactive phrases by the word "have" and proactive phrases by the word " can":

| HAVE LANGUAGE | "I CAN" LANGUAGE |
|---|---|
| I don't have the time. | I can make the time. |
| I have too many obligations. | I can set priorities. |
| I have no will power. | I can keep promises to myself. |

Becoming proactive has been difficult for me. I had listened to my childhood scripts, so deeply ingrained, all my life. If my children were sick, I had a right to be cranky. If my business partners ignored me, I had a right to ignore them. If my husband had a bad day, then, or course, I had a right to have a bad as well. I was convinced that my fate in life was in the hands of the unstable world around me, i.e., I was a victim of my circumstances. I was a textbook reactive. Not anymore.

As a human being I have the distinct power and freedom to "choose". This is not positive thinking; this goes far beyond positive thinking. I can choose to be proactive and become responsible for my life.

The realization that I am not a victim has "set me free". But being proactive requires constant vigilance on my part. Whenever I feel angry, sad, depressed, or out of control, I must remind myself to examine my language and refocus.

Recently I had a business relationship with partners end painfully. Rather than discuss the inevitable dissolution of the partnership, I was served with papers. I was deeply wounded and immediately took on the "victim" role. With the gently, kind and honest help of my husband and daughter, I recognized the old scripts. I then examined my reactive language: Why did they do this to me? How could they? Why are they out to get me? I then decided to change this language: "I can't control my feelings but I can choose my reactions to these feelings. Yes, my feelings are mine; it's ok to feel angry and hurt." But how I reacted to these feelings was, and is, a decision. I used visualization to change the way I viewed my partners and the way I viewed the ending of the business relationship. I visualized myself sitting with them when they wrote the letter. I began to see that they had no other tools at their disposal to end the relationship. It was an uncomfortable situation for them and they always dealt with uncomfortable situations in a very formal, businesslike manner. Emotion was not part of their repetoire.

In analyzing this event, I realized I was not a victim. I had simply not been proactive. Had I been proactive, the relationship would not have ended in such a painful way. I examined the last few months as partners and I realized that I too had practiced avoidance. In that realization, I wrote my business partners a letter thanking them for admitting to the obvious and taking the initiative. I also thanked them for the opportunity to have worked with them. They taught me a great deal about business.

In a strange way, this incident went from being painful, to comforting. I now realize that I will never revert back to being a reactive person (at least not for very long). The incident also made me aware of the wonderful support system I have developed. I now know I can always count on help from my wonderful family to remind me, when I temporarily fall back into the victim role, that I am not a victim. I am in charge of my life.

Take the time now to identify several difficult situations that you have experienced. Listen carefully to the phrases you use. List any reactive phrases below. Change these reactive phrases into proactive ones, and keep the list handy so that you can review it often.

| MY REACTIVE LANGUAGE: | MY PROACTIVE LANGUAGE: |
|---|---|
| _____ | _____ |
| _____ | _____ |
| _____ | _____ |
| _____ | _____ |
| _____ | _____ |
| _____ | _____ |

Now visualize yourself using these new proactive phrases. Actually visualize the situations that cause you to use reactive phrases and change those situations in your mind using positive, proactive phrases. Use great detail and visualize the situation many times; each time using your new proactive phrases. Now when that situation actually occurs you can implement your newly learned responses, rather than the old scripted ones.

New scripting is not easy. Remember to be kind to yourself. Recognizing the problem is the beginning of the solution.

# Step 2: Defining my roles-Who Am I?

Dr. Covey defines the word integrity as the ability to make promises to ourselves and keep them. How *wonderful;* I have integrity if I make promises to myself and if I keep those promises. In other words, it is actually selfish not to make my health a top priority. Without my health I can not fulfill my other roles in life. If I don't live each of my many roles I can not share my uniqueness with the world.

Successful people always work to maintain balance between their many varied roles. For example, I am a wife, mother, grandmother, daughter, sister, educator, business woman, roller blader, etc. If my sense of self worth comes from only one of these roles, I will not be effective nor will I be happy. To find true happiness I must work towards becoming effective in all areas of my life.

First and foremost, I am a human being. I must have a body to live in if I am to fulfill all of my other roles. Therefore, my role as a human being must supersede all other roles. The following is an outline of my roles in life:

### Dr. Jane's Roles:

HUMAN BEING
WOMAN
WIFE
MOTHER
GRANDMOTHER
DAUGHTER
SISTER
EDUCATOR
BUSINESS WOMAN
ROLLER BLADER
TENNIS PLAYER

I have given myself permission to be all of these individual parts. While this may sound easy, for many of us this is a huge step. I am a wife, yes. But I am also a mother and a business woman. Acknowledging all of these parts allows me the freedom to choose which parts I will concentrate on and when.

This decision to be "whole" has not changed what I do, per se. What it has done is change the way I view what I do. If I am being a business woman/educator I don't worry about being a wife. For example, if I am with a client at 8 o'clock in the evening and I am running late, I no longer worry about my husband at home getting hungry. In the first place, my husband is the greatest, easiest, mild mannered person I have ever known. He is also the most capable human being I have ever known. If he's hungry, he knows how to feed himself.

But, even if he were sitting home waiting for me to cook for him, my role as a business woman/educator at that moment supersedes my role as a "house-wife".

What being "whole" has done for me has taken the guilt out of my life. Defining my roles has allowed me the freedom to live each role in balance with the other roles. I now set weekly goals in each area, (see next section) and I make a commitment to myself to keep them. Of course, I allow for unexpected events. But once I have made a commitment to myself, I keep that commitment.

This next step is critical to your success, not only in health, but in all areas of your life. Don't take any shortcuts. Take the time now to identify your roles and give yourself permission to be "whole". Remember, we are a combination of all our roles, all that we do, and all that we want to do.

```
┌─────────────────────────────────────────────────────────────┐
│                        MY ROLES                               │
│                                                               │
│   1. Human Being:        2. _____      3. _____     │
│                                                               │
│                                                               │
│   4. _____          5. _____      6. _____     │
│                                                               │
│                                                               │
│   7. _____          8. _____      9. _____     │
│                                                               │
│   I give myself permission to be all of these roles.  The    │
│   combination of these roles is what makes me unique, and I   │
│   have decided to share my unique-                            │
│   ness with the world.                                        │
│                                                               │
│                    _____          │
│                         Signature              Date           │
└─────────────────────────────────────────────────────────────┘
```

\Now that you have identified all of your roles, be sure to give yourself permission to live all of your parts and beome whole.

Time is not the critical factor here. If you are a mother of young children you will obviously spend more time in that role. The important point is to take **some** time to fulfill all your roles. As a grandmother with grandchildren that live thousands of miles away, my goal many weeks is as simple as calling them to tell them how much I love them. On the other hand, my role as a business woman and educator takes up most of my time.

If you are centered on one role to the exclusion of others, ask yourself why? Are there old scripts from your past preventing you from living the other roles? If so, take the time right now to rewrite the scripts.

# Step 3: How Do I Want My Story to End?

Now that you have identified your roles and are working on changing the old reactive scripts to new proactive ones, it's time to evaluate "Your Story". In his book, Dr. Covey describes this next step as "keeping the end in mind". This step asks the question: "How do I want to be remembered by the people I care about and the people I share my life with?" "What do I want them to say about me when my story is ended?" This is very different from worrying about what other people think of me. In this step I am asking myself "how I do I want to be remembered". To answer this question I must search deep within myself and examine what my real values are.

For me, this step was (and is) very powerful and life changing. I initially visualized my grown children while writing the end of my story. I wanted them to remember their mom as "loving them unconditionally and always being there for them when they needed her". I wanted them to have memories of me comforting them when they were disappointed in themselves, or when the world seemed unkind, cold, or scary. I wanted to be remembered for providing kind non-judgmental advice, not criticizing or judging. I wanted them to recount how they were able to pick up the phone anytime and know that they would have a loving, caring, honest, Mom on the other end of the line. I wanted them to believe no one could ever love them as much and as unconditionally as their Mom did.

In many ways this visualization was comforting. I was already doing many of the things I wanted to be remembered for. Years ago my husband and I decided to handle everyday decisions regarding our children by visualizing ourselves in our 100's (it use to be our 80's) sitting in our rocking chairs looking back on the very decisions we were about to make. Because of this visualization we handled the everyday decisions from a more realistic, global perspective.

The painful part came when I examined the end of my story in context of my role as a business woman and a wife. As a business woman I realized I was not acting/reacting in a manner that I wanted to be remembered for. I needed to rewrite my script; a script that I am constantly working on.

I also realized that my role as a wife needed rescripting. I pride myself on possessing the attribute of treasuring all people for their uniqueness. My visualization as a wife made me realize that there were times when I was not viewing my wonderful husband with this same philosophy.

Rewriting this script was actually easier and less painful than I had imagined. I found the process of writing the end of my story on how I wanted my husband to remember me very "liberating". I wanted him to tell the world that his wife was a wonderful business woman, staying until after 8 p.m. with clients, because she truly cared about their success in health. I also knew that I would certainly not want (and I know he would not want) him to recount how I rushed home to cook his dinner at the expense of these clients. From our many conversations, I knew he would recount all the times we spent traveling and how well we "traveled together". I also knew he would recount how much I loved my children and what a wonderful grandmother I was. But most importantly (and I had lost track of this in the craziness of our hectic lives) I visualized him recounting how much I loved him "just as he is"; how I always laughed at his stupid jokes; and how perfect we were for each other.

Implementing this new script was easy. I hadn't realized that when I gave myself permission to be whole, I had automatically given my husband permission to be whole. I can now love him for the special human being he is without the old strings attached.

Take a look at your roles again. Picture each role and how you want to be remembered by each key person, or persons involved in that role. Find a quiet place where you can be alone with your thoughts, and visualize each role individually. If the process is painful, you may want to visualize only one role today, or this week, and proceed to the next role tomorrow, or next week.

Begin with your role as a human being - man or woman and ask yourself how you want to be remembered.

MY ROLES

1. Human Being:

How do I want to be remembered by _____

_____

_____

2. _____:

How do I want to be remembered by _____

_____

_____

3. _____:

How do I want to be remembered by _____

_____

_____

4. _____:

How do I want to be remembered by _____

_____

_____ _____

5. _____:

How do I want to be remembered by _____

_____

_____

If you have followed these steps, and have truly "searched your soul, you can no longer remain a reactive person. You are well on your way to taking charge of your life.

**Congratulations!**

# Step 4: Putting It Into Practice

Now that you have identified your roles, given yourself permission to be "all of your parts", and written the end of your story, its time to put it all into practice.

This step is learning to live your uniqueness by making promises to yourself and keeping them. In this step you need to list two or three important results you wish to accomplish in each area of your life. Remember to keep it simple. Do not allow yourself to become overwhelmed.

At this point, begin with your role as a human being. You can progress to your other roles later.

**I challenge you to a 6 week life-changing program**. This challenge requires dedication and fortitude on your part. For the next 6 weeks I challenge you to make small commitments to yourself and keep them. Begin with small changes; ones that you can live with and are relatively easy to accomplish. Don't set a goal of exercising 30 minutes every day for the next 7 days if you are not exercising at all right now. You will set yourself up to fail, and the whole process will simply reinforce your reactive responses; i.e., I knew I couldn't do it.

Perhaps your goal may be as simple as walking to and from your car parked at the furthermost point in the parking lot. Great! You can then progress to climbing the stairs etc.

Your goal in the next 6 weeks may be to become an active person by walking. Great! You can progress to 10 minutes per day for 3 out of 7 days; and ultimately work towards your goal of walking 10 minutes per day 5 out of 7 days.

Perhaps your goal is to reduce cholesterol levels by limiting your saturated fat intake. Great! Follow the same process. Begin by cutting down on one of your favorite saturated fatty foods, i.e., I'll have a hamburger every other day instead of every day.

# Step 5: Hints on Setting Goals

The following are hints on setting goals. Remember, make small, easy to accomplish goals at first and work your way into more difficult ones.

## Setting Goals must follow the S M A R T rule.

S stands for specific — The goal must be specific. If the goal is too broad it will be beyond achievement.

M stands for measurable — The goal must be measurable. One can set goals, but if they are not measurable there is no way of knowing if that goal has been achieved.

A stands for value — The goal must be important and of value to you. If it isn't important to you then the goal will not be accomplished. For example, if a spouse wants you to lose weight, the first time you get mad at your spouse   you will overeat "to get even".

R stands for realistic — The goal must be realistic. If you are not exercising now, it is unrealistic to set a goal of exercising one hour everyday. You will become discouraged and give up on the goal altogether.

T stands for Time — All goals must have a deadline. If no deadline exists, there is no incentive to achieve the goal.

# Step 6: Goals For Health

OK. Are You Ready? Start off initially by looking at setting long term goals. Use the following table to organize your thoughts. List two results you wish to accomplish (always keeping in mind your ultimate goal of how you want your story to end). These goals will need to be occasionally revised and reviewed. Above all, if you feel overwhelmed, take one step at a time. One small step is better than none. One small goal accomplished builds self-esteem and confidence. Many "sincere" large goals failed destroy self-esteem and confidence.

# Long Range Health Goals

Within one year I will:

Goal 1: _____

_____

_____

_____

_____

_____

_____

_____

Goal 2: _____

_____

_____

_____

_____

_____

_____

Now transform these long range goals into short range goals which are still reasonable, measurable, specific, etc. What is it that you wish to accomplish in each role in the next 6 weeks, keeping in mind your long range goals.

•

# My 6 week Goals

By the end of six weeks I will:

Goal 1: _____

_____

_____

_____

_____

_____

_____

_____

Goal 2: _____

_____

_____

_____

_____

_____

_____

Now that you have identified what it is you will do in the next 6 weeks, use the following calendar and specifically identify the daily tasks required to accomplish your goals.

For example, if your goal is to begin an exercise program and reduce your cholesterol levels, you can plan your weekly calendar accordingly. Set aside time each week to accomplish your goal for exercise and write yourself notes on which days you will have the hamburger, etc. At the end of the week, you can review the calendar to see if you have accomplished the tasks you set. While this process is arduous and time consuming it produces the wanted results - you will have become a proactive person in charge of your own life.

If you find yourself making excuses, write down the language you use and rewrite the script to proactive language. If necessary go back to step 1.

# Your Six Week Challenge

How to use the following pages:

1. Identify one or two goals you wish to accomplish to reach your six week health goals.

2. Use the calendar on the weekly pages to identify times in which you can perform the tasks necessary to attain your goals.

Remember, there's no hurry. Success isn't in how much you do in 6 weeks. Success is in completing what you say you will do, no matter what it is.

**Good Luck and Don't Give Up! The life you save is your own!** Each commitment you keep is one small step towards taking charge of your health. Remember, mankind needs you to share your uniqueness with the world.

# Week 1
# My Roles

By the end of this week I will:

Goal 1: _____

_____

_____

_____

_____

_____

_____

_____


Goal 2: _____

_____

_____

_____

_____

_____

_____

_____

# Week 1 Calendar

|          | Sun | Mon | Tue | Wed | Thu | Fri | Sat |
|----------|-----|-----|-----|-----|-----|-----|-----|
| 7 a.m.   |     |     |     |     |     |     |     |
| 8 a.m.   |     |     |     |     |     |     |     |
| 9 a.m.   |     |     |     |     |     |     |     |
| 10 a.m.  |     |     |     |     |     |     |     |
| 11 a.m.  |     |     |     |     |     |     |     |
| 12 a.m.  |     |     |     |     |     |     |     |
| 1 p.m.   |     |     |     |     |     |     |     |
| 2 p.m.   |     |     |     |     |     |     |     |
| 3 p.m.   |     |     |     |     |     |     |     |
| 4 p.m.   |     |     |     |     |     |     |     |
| 5 p.m.   |     |     |     |     |     |     |     |
| 6 p.m.   |     |     |     |     |     |     |     |
| 7-10 p.m.|     |     |     |     |     |     |     |

# Week 2
## My Roles

By the end of this week I will:

Goal 1: _____

_____

_____

_____

_____

_____

_____

_____

Goal 2: _____

_____

_____

_____

_____

_____

_____

_____

# Week 2 Calendar

|          | Sun | Mon | Tue | Wed | Thu | Fri | Sat |
|----------|-----|-----|-----|-----|-----|-----|-----|
| 7 a.m.   |     |     |     |     |     |     |     |
| 8 a.m.   |     |     |     |     |     |     |     |
| 9 a.m.   |     |     |     |     |     |     |     |
| 10 a.m.  |     |     |     |     |     |     |     |
| 11 a.m.  |     |     |     |     |     |     |     |
| 12 a.m.  |     |     |     |     |     |     |     |
| 1 p.m.   |     |     |     |     |     |     |     |
| 2 p.m.   |     |     |     |     |     |     |     |
| 3 p.m.   |     |     |     |     |     |     |     |
| 4 p.m.   |     |     |     |     |     |     |     |
| 5 p.m.   |     |     |     |     |     |     |     |
| 6 p.m.   |     |     |     |     |     |     |     |
| 7-10 p.m.|     |     |     |     |     |     |     |

# Week 3
# My Roles

By the end of this week I will:

Goal 1: _____

_____

_____

_____

_____

_____

_____

_____

Goal 2: _____

_____

_____

_____

_____

_____

_____

_____

# Week 3 Calendar

| | Sun | Mon | Tue | Wed | Thu | Fri | Sat |
|---|---|---|---|---|---|---|---|
| 7 a.m. | | | | | | | |
| 8 a.m. | | | | | | | |
| 9 a.m. | | | | | | | |
| 10 a.m. | | | | | | | |
| 11 a.m. | | | | | | | |
| 12 a.m. | | | | | | | |
| 1 p.m. | | | | | | | |
| 2 p.m. | | | | | | | |
| 3 p.m. | | | | | | | |
| 4 p.m. | | | | | | | |
| 5 p.m. | | | | | | | |
| 6 p.m. | | | | | | | |
| 7-10 p.m. | | | | | | | |

# Week 4
## My Roles

By the end of this week I will:

Goal 1: _____

_____

_____

_____

_____

_____

_____

_____

Goal 2: _____

_____

_____

_____

_____

_____

_____

_____

# Week 4 Calendar

|          | Sun | Mon | Tue | Wed | Thu | Fri | Sat |
|----------|-----|-----|-----|-----|-----|-----|-----|
| 7 a.m.   |     |     |     |     |     |     |     |
| 8 a.m.   |     |     |     |     |     |     |     |
| 9 a.m.   |     |     |     |     |     |     |     |
| 10 a.m.  |     |     |     |     |     |     |     |
| 11 a.m.  |     |     |     |     |     |     |     |
| 12 a.m.  |     |     |     |     |     |     |     |
| 1 p.m.   |     |     |     |     |     |     |     |
| 2 p.m.   |     |     |     |     |     |     |     |
| 3 p.m.   |     |     |     |     |     |     |     |
| 4 p.m.   |     |     |     |     |     |     |     |
| 5 p.m.   |     |     |     |     |     |     |     |
| 6 p.m.   |     |     |     |     |     |     |     |
| 7-10 p.m.|     |     |     |     |     |     |     |

# Week 5
## My Roles

By the end of this week I will:

Goal 1: _____

_____

_____

_____

_____

_____

_____

_____


Goal 2: _____

_____

_____

_____

_____

_____

_____

_____

# Week 5 Calendar

| | Sun | Mon | Tue | Wed | Thu | Fri | Sat |
|---|---|---|---|---|---|---|---|
| 7 a.m. | | | | | | | |
| 8 a.m. | | | | | | | |
| 9 a.m. | | | | | | | |
| 10 a.m. | | | | | | | |
| 11 a.m. | | | | | | | |
| 12 a.m. | | | | | | | |
| 1 p.m. | | | | | | | |
| 2 p.m. | | | | | | | |
| 3 p.m. | | | | | | | |
| 4 p.m. | | | | | | | |
| 5 p.m. | | | | | | | |
| 6 p.m. | | | | | | | |
| 7-10 p.m. | | | | | | | |

# Week 6
# My Roles

By the end of this week I will:

Goal 1: _____

_____

_____

_____

_____

_____

_____

_____


Goal 2: _____

_____

_____

_____

_____

_____

_____

_____

# Week 6 Calendar

| | Sun | Mon | Tue | Wed | Thu | Fri | Sat |
|---|---|---|---|---|---|---|---|
| 7 a.m. | | | | | | | |
| 8 a.m. | | | | | | | |
| 9 a.m. | | | | | | | |
| 10 a.m. | | | | | | | |
| 11 a.m. | | | | | | | |
| 12 a.m. | | | | | | | |
| 1 p.m. | | | | | | | |
| 2 p.m. | | | | | | | |
| 3 p.m. | | | | | | | |
| 4 p.m. | | | | | | | |
| 5 p.m. | | | | | | | |
| 6 p.m. | | | | | | | |
| 7-10 p.m. | | | | | | | |

# The six week challenge is over.

How did you do?  How about another six week challenge?

Please let me know if the preceding challenge helped you take charge of your health.

I hope to hear from you! Send suggestions, stories, etc. to Dr. Jane at info@lifestylemanagement.com

Now write yourself a congratulatory letter. Review whenever you need a lift, and remember you can always perform an encore.

_____

_____

_____

_____

_____

_____

_____

_____

_____

_____

_____

_____

_____

_____

_____

_____

_____

_____

_____

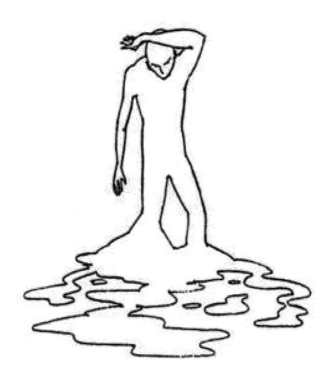

# Part III
# The Basics

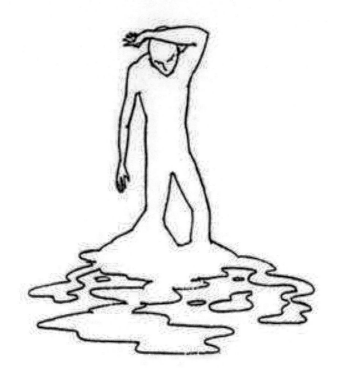

# Chapter 1
# Nutrition Basics

# Nutrition Basics

The diet industry is a $54 billion industry with a 95% fail rate. Diets are a big fat lie. Despite all our "diet foods" we are still getting fatter. Despite all the money spent yearly on dieting, 66 percent of Americans are overweight today compared to 58 percent in 1983. If this weight increase were considered a disease, it would be an epidemic.

So why doesn't dieting work? All diets look at scale weight. The following objects weigh the same.

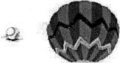

Weight does not determine size. Read the following sections carefully and learn how to become the hard ball - not the beach ball.

## Nutrition Essentials

Without food you will die! If you become deficient in essential nutrients, parts of your body will not function well. If the deficiency continues, parts of your body will cease to function, and then eventually you will die. That's what essential means - essential to stay alive. Some essential nutrients provide your body with energy; these nutrients are carbohydrates, fats, and proteins. Vitamins and minerals, while they do not provide energy, have other roles that are just as vital. Let's start off by learning about the energy nutrients.

## About Carbs

Did you know your body needs carbs (glucose) and oxygen to burn fat? Your muscles use fat in conjunction with glucose and oxygen. How much fat your muscles can utilize depends on how much muscle you have, how much oxygen reaches your muscles and the process requires glucose. So an aerobically fit person with lots of muscle (and glucose stored in muscle) burns much more fat than an aerobically unfit person. Your muscles and liver store glucose for you. If your muscles run out of glucose they cannot utilize fat for energy—no matter how much fat is stored in your fat cells.

What does this mean for you? It means that you must eat to burn fat. You must begin your day by eating breakfast. Breakfast fuels your muscles and readies them to burn fat. A word of caution: your muscles can store only a finite amount of carbs, so it is much better to eat smaller portions and to eat more frequently during the day. Overeating at one meal forces the body to store (beyond what it can store in the muscle and liver) the excess carb calories as fat in the fat cell.

The above facts are crucial to lifelong weight management. People who don't eat increase the percentage of fat stored in their bodies. Consider this: anorexics weighing 80 to 90 pounds can have as much as 40 to 50 percent body fat. Eventually they die because their hearts and liver "shrivel" up. Many of us have been taught that not eating will make us slim, but in truth, if you do not eat, your muscle mass will decrease and you will actually become fatter. (Turn to Table 1 at the end of this chapter for a list of foods that are good sources of carbohydrates.)

Bottom line: Eat carbs to help you burn fat. Yes, too many carbs will eventually be stored as fat, but you have storage depots other than fat cells that can be filled first. So don't be afraid to eat small amounts of carbs when you are hungry.

# About Fat

Fats are sometimes confusing. You've heard about saturated fats, unsaturated fats, and cholesterol. Which is the good fat? Which is the bad fat? The most important point to remember is that fat from animal products (palm oil and coconut oil as well) are the fats that increase your risk for heart disease and are also the types of fats that are stored in your fat cells. When you eat beef or butter, the fat goes to your fat cells to be stored and, on the way there, clogs your arteries. These fats must be moderated in your diet or you will never be successful in health or weight management. Notice I said "moderated." It doesn't mean you can never have these foods, it simply means that you must choose to have them less often.

The fats found in oils (flax, olive, canola), seeds (flax,soy,walnuts,etc.), and fish, have very important roles in the body. These fats ( phospholipids) contain essential fatty acids which are involved in immune function, membrane function, and many other roles. In other words, you need small amounts of these fats in your diet. Notice that I said "small." So what happens if you cook your dinner with a quarter cup of olive oil (60 grams of fat)? True, this oil will not clog your arteries, but this amount is far too much; your body will take the excess and store it in your fat cells, just like the animal fats. (Turn to Table 2 at the end of this chapter for a list of good and bad fats.)

Bottom line: Begin to add small amounts of the "good" foods every day to your diet. Begin to decrease red meat, cream, butter, margarine, and cheese.

# About Protein

Protein is vital for every reaction in your body. The fact that you can see (vision) is due to protein, the fact that your muscles move is due to proteins, your immune system is dependent on proteins, and growth hormone and insulin are also proteins. Proteins are anabolic - they are necessary to build muscle, precious muscle that utilizes calories.

Since proteins have so many vital roles, it is very "expensive" to use them for energy. In order for your body to use proteins for energy, it must take the amino acids that make up proteins and turn some of them into glucose. These amino acids have an element, called nitrogen, which is toxic and must be eliminated by your liver and kidneys. Hence, ingesting excess protein is not wise. At best, excess protein taxes your liver and kidneys; at worst, it can cause deficiencies of other nutrients and can cause permanent liver damage. (Turn to Table 3 at the end of this chapter for a list of foods that are good sources of protein.)

Bottom line: Adequate amounts of protein in your daily diet are necessary for all the vital roles of proteins, which include building muscle when doing resistance training. Excess simply taxes the liver and is stored as fat.

## About Vitamins and Minerals

Vitamins and minerals do not provide energy for your body. They do, however, have many vital roles, one of which is to help "pull" energy from carbohydrates. So if you do not include fruits, vegetables, and whole grains in your diet, you will be exhausted, even if you eat enough of the other carbs.

Certain vitamins, known as antioxidants (Vitamins A, C, and E) have been shown to decrease your risk for all forms of cancer, heart disease, cataracts, and other chronic diseases.

Bottom line: If you want to do everything in your power to stave off disease, you need lots of fruits and vegetables. How much? People who exercise need seven to nine servings a day. Don't panic. It's easier than you think. A glass of orange juice, a banana for a snack, a large salad with lunch (not just iceberg lettuce), and a cup of vegetables at dinner adds up to eight servings. (Turn to Table 4 at the end of this chapter for an explanation of serving size.)

## About Exercise

Health and lifelong weight management must incorporate both healthy eating and exercise (See Fig. 1). Even if you eat perfectly all your life, if you do not exercise you will get fatter as you age. Why? If you do not exercise aerobically on a regular basis you will lose aerobic capacity (the capacity to burn fat efficiently), resulting in increased body fat. If you do not perform muscle strengthening exercises on a regular basis you will lose muscle (precious muscle that stores and utilizes calories) also resulting in increased body fat.

How much exercise is necessary? The important question is not just how much exercise, but at what intensity? Also equally important is how the exercise should be performed. This book will address the components of exercise in another chapter. For now you must understand that healthy eating is only half the picture. You must incorporate cardiovascular, muscle strengthening, and flexibility exercises into your lifestyle if you are to maintain health and weight management throughout your life.

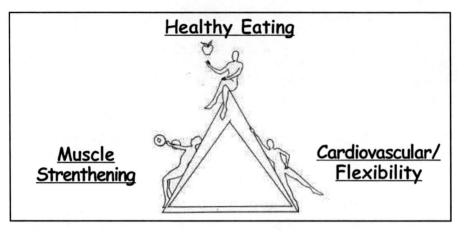

**Healthy Eating**

**Muscle Strenthening**

**Cardiovascular/ Flexibility**

Bottom line: Your body fat will increase if you don't exercise, even if you eat healthy.

## About Aging

The data is in! We know how to slow the aging process, and even how to reverse it. Sound good? Read on.

Researchers at Tufts University have discarded the chronological approach to aging. As people age the diversity in physiological parameters increases immensely. Have you noticed how some 70 and 80 year olds look more like 50 and 60 year olds, and some 50 year olds look more like 90 year olds? This phenomenon occurs not only cosmetically, but physiologically as well. Some of us over 50 are biologically more similar to 30 and 40 year olds. YEA!

The most important parameters of staying younger physiologically include aerobic capacity, muscle mass, muscle strength, and percent body fat (sound familiar). Muscle, to a far greater extent than people realize, is responsible for slowing the aging process. A high muscle to fat ratio causes metabolism to rise allowing the body to burn more fat, hence making it easier to keep the weight off. The more muscle I have, the more calories can be stored in these muscles (instead of as fat in fat cells) and the more fat burning machinery to utilize calories. Also, the more aerobically fit I am the more efficient my body is at burning fat.

Exercising not only helps us feel younger and have more energy, it reduces our chances for diabetes, heart disease, high blood pressure, and osteoporosis. Everyone should exercise. So no excuses we all must exercise.

Studies have confirmed if you eat your fruits and vegetables, your chances for all forms of cancer are also decreased (see section on supplements). Healthy eating is a matter of changing slowly. For example, if you drink whole milk now, go to 2% milk not skim milk. Once you have adjusted to 2% milk, then try 1% milk. When 1% milk tastes good to you, try skim milk.

Do you need any more reasons to add two or three exercise sessions per week to your lifestyle and add some fruits and vegetables to your diet? I don't.

## About the Scale

If you have been a "dieter" in the past, you must be patient, and don't get on a scale! The following story about Mike will illustrate why the scale is your enemy.

Mike is a 55-year-old executive trying desperately to win the battle of the bulge. He steps on the scale every morning to monitor his weight. At six foot, two inches and 200 pounds, he doesn't look "overweight." But Mike is frustrated. He eats less (by skipping lunch) and exercises more in order to keep his weight from creeping up, but he now buys clothes a size larger. He is always tired and hungry, and often cranky.

The scale is deceiving Mike. The scale only measures his total mass - 200 pounds. In Figure 2, Mike is shown as he is at 200 pounds. Figure 3 shows Mike's "twin" who, at the same height and weight, is leaner and in better condition. The question the scale answers for Mike is, "How much do I weigh?" It cannot answer the more important question, "How much of that 200 pounds is calorie-burning muscle versus metabolically inactive fat?" Therefore, the scale provides an unreliable "picture" of Mike's true condition.

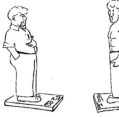

Figure 2          Figure 3
Mike              Mike's Twin

Mike, like millions of Americans, believes his body is burning fat when he does not eat, but the truth of the matter is that by following his low-calorie regimen, he is actually losing muscle at a rate equal to or greater than his loss of fat.

The body relies primarily on carbohydrates for energy. If the body runs out of carbohydrates, it cannot burn fat; it is then forced to break down muscle into its constituent amino acids, some of which can make carbohydrates for us. Fats cannot make carbohydrates for us.

Low calorie diets force the body to utilize lean muscle, the biggest user of fats, for energy; that precious muscle that burns calories is being broken down to provide the energy needed to keep Mike going through his day. To regain the lost muscle, Mike needs to eat healthy and incorporate muscle-strengthening exercises into his exercise program. He also needs to understand a few basic facts about how his body uses calories.

To end this vicious cycle of eating less and increasing his body fat, Mike must fuel his muscles with adequate amounts of carbohydrates every day. He must be sure to limit the fat in his diet and incorporate adequate amounts of protein. So where does Mike start? How can he, and millions of Americans like him, break the cycle?

Mike can start to break the cycle by first adding a good carbohydrate source to his breakfast. A bagel or cereal is a much better choice than Mike's regular breakfast of coffee and a croissant. A croissant contains more fat calories than carbohydrate calories and will not provide enough carbohydrates to fuel Mike's body for the morning. To complete his breakfast, he should add a protein source such as milk or yogurt.

Mike should also incorporate a few muscle strengthening exercises into his daily routine (push-ups and squats are a good start). When Mike has mastered these changes and made them a part of his lifestyle, he can continue to make more changes.

The next goal for Mike should be to eat a healthy, low-fat lunch. If he skips lunch, his body will turn to his muscles for "fuel" and run on muscle energy all afternoon. When he finally sits down to eat at 8:00 p.m., exhausted, stressed and starving, he will most likely overeat. Overeating at night forces the body to store excess calories as fat, even if those calories are carbohydrates.

Lunch should include a good carbohydrate choice, a low-fat protein choice and a fruit or salad. A change to his evening eating patterns will be the most difficult for Mike. He should not attempt these changes until he has mastered breakfast and lunch.

Mike will face many obstacles and challenges while making these lifestyle changes. Advertising and nutritional labeling, designed to aid Mike in making proper choices, will confuse him. For example, 1 percent milk is 18 percent fat by calories. Margarine that claims to be totally fat-free is actually 100 percent fat (one tablespoon of Promise Ultra Fat Free Margarine has five calories per tablespoon and contains five calories from fat).

Mike will also face friendly saboteurs. Friends, and even family members, will try to coax Mike into eating eggs and bacon for breakfast or will offer him a donut. It's no wonder people like Mike give up before they even try.

My advice to Mike, and to all of you, is don't give up; make one small change at a time. Make that change realistic and obtainable. Work on incorporating a healthy breakfast for one or two weeks. Once that becomes habit, work on lunch alternatives. Continue to set new goals for yourself. Remember, as Chinese philosopher Lao Tzu wrote, "a journey of a thousand miles starts where your feet stand." This is a journey best made one step at a time.

The benefits are well worth the effort. There is a direct relationship between the quality of food we eat, our physical activity level and long-term health. While there are no guarantees, if Mike changes his lifestyle his chances of getting these diseases will be greatly decreased. Not only will Mike feel better, he'll look better, and he will also have more energy to enjoy his later years. His approaching retirement can be viewed as another exciting stage in life in which to fulfill all his dreams rather than a final stage of life to be dreaded. Remember, we are responsible for our health and the quality of our lives, even through our senior years. We must all leave this world one day, but how and when we do is partially in our control.

# About Cholesterol

Cholesterol is a fat that we obtain from our diets and that our bodies also manufacture. Cholesterol has important roles; it is the precursor molecule for testosterone, estrogen, and bile acids. Cholesterol, along with sunlight, provides us with vitamin D.

An excess or deficiency of cholesterol can cause disease. Excess cholesterol increases our risk for all forms of cardiovascular disease. A deficiency can lead to decreased estrogen in women. Young women on very low-fat diets have been found to have decreased levels of estrogen; in some cases they become amenorrheic.

Much research is being done on cholesterol biochemistry. To summarize what we know about lowering blood cholesterol levels:

Reduce total dietary fat. Saturated fat is a bigger culprit than dietary cholesterol. Reducing total fat intake to 10 percent of total caloric intake is ideal, although very difficult. Dr. Dean Ornish of the University of San Francisco School of Medicine has had excellent results in not only reducing heart disease, but in actually reversing it with a very low-fat diet (10 percent of total caloric intake). This diet contains no added oils, eliminates caffeine totally, and incorporates moderate exercise and stress management. Dr. Ornish's diet is a severely restricted diet; however, for someone who has already had a heart attack the other options are far less attractive. For the rest of us, a dietary intake of 20 percent total fat is recommended with at least 10 percent unsaturated fat.

Reduce dietary cholesterol. Reducing cholesterol intake from 500 to 200 milligrams a day will lower total blood cholesterol by an average of ten milligrams. The response varies; some people have little response while others have greater response.

Include lots of fiber, which is found in oats, beans, fruits and vegetables. Oats have a fiber-rich bran layer that effectively lowers cholesterol; beans, fruits and vegetables have also been shown to have cholesterol-lowering properties.

Eat more fish. The oilier fish, such as salmon, mackerel, albacore, and herring, guard against heart disease and hypertension. Eating two to three meals of fish per week will reduce your risk of heart disease.

Add small amounts of olive oil to your diet. Olive oil has been shown to be heart-healthy. Small amounts of olive oil have been shown to decrease LDL cholesterol while preserving HDL (the good) cholesterol. Cooking with olive oil may not be as good as adding uncooked oil to your foods because cooking with olive oil decreases some of its antioxidant properties.

Include soy protein in your diet. A New England Journal of Medicine study found that when people ate soy protein rather than animal protein, their cholesterol and LDL cholesterol levels were significantly reduced. HDL was unaffected.

Decrease caffeine in your diet. Caffeine has been shown to increase cholesterol levels.

Minimize concentrated simple sugars. Concentrated simple sugars and other concentrated sweeteners, such as fructose, corn syrup, and honey, lead to the production of a liver enzyme (HMG-CoA reductase) that causes the liver to make more cholesterol. Hence, eating sugar can increase your blood cholesterol levels.

## About Stress

What is stress? Stress was originally defined as the "nonspecific response of the body to any demand made upon it." Stress is caused by a stressor or a stimulus that has the potential for causing the fight or flight response. The body responds to stress with an elaborate series of physiological steps using the nervous and hormone systems to bring about defensive readiness in every part of the body. The heart beats faster, breathing changes, blood pressure increases, serum cholesterol increases, more acid is secreted in the stomach, and muscle proteins are broken down into their constituent amino acids.

Some of these amino acids are transported to the liver and made into glucose which is poured into the bloodstream readying the body to run or fight. Liver glycogen is also being broken down into glucose when fighting or running begins. Under chronic psychological stress the muscles are not able to take up these nutrients; these stress products build up in the bloodstream and increase the risk of development of chronic diseases such as diabetes, cardiovascular disease, hypertension, etc.

The experts tell us that in order to reduce stress you must:

1. Recognize the stressors—are they routine or unique?

2. Recognize your reaction to stress (physically and psychologically).

3. Recognize how you cope.

4. Determine how you can cope in a better way.

5. Learn to relax.

Many people eat when stressed, while others are unable to eat. Both situations are detrimental to health. In a recent article in Health magazine, Susan Kayman, a health educator, studied women who had successfully maintained long term weight loss. She observed that the biggest obstacle to permanent weight loss was not the lack of willpower, but the lack of time. Successful "losers" shop, plan, and cook; they are good at organization and problem solving. If you are a stress eater you need to get organized, plan meals ahead, have low calorie healthy snacks available, and always shop with a list. If you are a stress non-eater, you also need to plan and have healthy foods available and visible to remind you to eat.

Remember stress is a response. According to Jerrod Greenberg, author of Comprehensive Stress Management, "You are in much greater control of you than you ever realized....Managing stress is really just exercising that control, rather than giving it up to others or to your environment....You may not be able to get other people to change what they say or do, but certainly you can change how you react to what they say or do."

**You are in charge of you.**

Bottom Line: Stress is catabolic, that is it breaks down muscle tissue. People under high stress will have a more difficult time building muscle.

# About Supplements

Do I recommend taking supplements? The answer is "YES, BUT!" I recommend a multiple vitamin, however only as an insurance policy for those days when you don't eat enough fruits or vegetables.

For women who do not get enough calcium in their diet, I also recommend calcium supplements. The recommendation for adequate calcium intake is four servings of dairy per day, about 1200 mg of calcium. If dairy products are lacking in your diet, the best and easiest way to obtain calcium is simply by taking a Tums with meals. Each Tums tablet can provide you with approximately 200 to 400 mg of calcium (read the label).

Bottom Line: The latest research shows that vitamin pills are not equivalent to eating fruits and vegetables. Studies show that subjects who incorporated pills into their diets did not show decreased risk for chronic disease, only those who ate the real thing - fruits and vegetables - did. Recent studies have indicated that certain foods, such as fruits and vegetables, contain over 200 phytochemicals that also have antioxidant properties.

# More About Supplements

There are many vitamin companies trying to convince the American public that it is necessary to ingest huge amounts of these micronutrients to stay healthy. Micronutrient supplements are big business, so beware of false claims. Research suggests that certain nutrients, such as antioxidants, do reduce our risk for all forms of cancer and perhaps heart disease; however, the amounts needed are not excessive amounts.

An excess of any of these micronutrients can be as detrimental to health as a deficiency. Some of the same diseases caused by deficiencies of nutrients are also caused by the consumption of excessive amounts of those same nutrients. Toxicity levels differ for each nutrient. Ten times the RDA for Vitamin D is toxic. Persons taking 3000 mg or more of vitamin C get scurvy if they discontinue taking the vitamin. Therefore, it is unwise to take supplements that contain large amounts of micronutrients, and if large amounts are taken it is wise to reduce the amount slowly as with some drugs.

Bottom line: People should not be fooled into thinking that they can take a pill every day and never have to eat a fruit or vegetable ever again in order to be healthy.

# About Science

Are you looking for miracle drugs to build muscle, burn fat, or replace healthy eating. If you are, you may very likely be "drawn in" by any and all marketing schemes. How can you differentiate between these marketing schemes (that appear scientific) and sound nutrition research that can be trusted? Here are some questions you need to ask to assess the accuracy of any new health claims:

1. **What is the study design?**

2. **What are the limitations associated with this type of study?**

3. **Was the research published in a peer-reviewed journal?** Peer review refers to the process by which the editors of a journal ask experts in a study's subject to review the study (usually 7 to 10 other experts) to ensure it was conducted appropriately. If the study was poorly designed or comes up short, it is usually not published.

Dr. Sears (The Zone Diet) makes claims about research that he has completed, but his research has never been published in any journal—peer reviewed or otherwise.

4. **How was the study conducted? What was the sample size and duration of the study?** If a study reports that the tested product builds muscle in animals, it should not be assumed that the same results will be seen in humans. Studies reporting results seen on very small populations for short time periods may not be reliable.

Clenbuterol, a beta-agonist was shown to build muscle in growing animals. Wow! People in Europe jumped on the band wagon. In later studies, clenbuterol in adult animals was shown to store fat, not build muscle. In humans, clenbuterol turned out to be a killer. Humans have beta receptors, not only on fat and muscle cells, but also heart cells and clenbuterol entering heart cells kills. One study (Long-term oral creatine supplementation does not impair renal function in healthy athletes) boasts no ill effects of oral creatine supplementation. However, only two, young, healthy athletes made it to five years. Are you convinced that there are no long term effects based on only two people? (Med.Sci.Sports Exerc. vol 31(8)1108-10.1999)?

5. **Who paid for the study?** Was the study funded by the same company that sells the product being touted as a new life saving discovery? Many studies reporting positive muscle building effects of creatine phosphate were of short duration with very few people. Most studies were funded by the manufacturers of the product.

6. **Was there a control group?** To obtain reliable data, the study should be a controlled double blind study in which the subjects (and persons actually involved in distributing the product) are not informed as to whether they are given the actual product being tested or a placebo. Without a control group, there is no way of knowing if the product is actually producing the wanted results or if other variables within the group caused the wanted results.

Placebo effect is the measurable, observable, or felt improvement in health not attributable to treatment. Some believe the placebo effect is psychological, due to a belief in the treatment or to a subjective feeling of improvement. In other words, if people believe a product will work, there is a distinct possibility that it will. In a study of 17 asthmatics, some subjects experienced a temporary decline in lung function after breathing in a solution that they were told would make breathing more difficult but was, in fact, ordinary saline solution. According to the researchers it is common to find a placebo effect of 30% or more in people with asthma[1].

Dr. Irving Kirsch, a psychologist at the University of Connecticut, analyzed 39 studies, done between 1974 and 1995, of depressed patients treated with drugs, psychotherapy, or a combination of both. He found that 50% of the drug effect is due to the placebo response[2].

Fifty-two percent of colitis patients treated with a placebo in 11 different trials reported feeling better - and 50% of the inflamed intestines actually looked better when assessed with a sigmoidoscope[3].

When placebos are given for pain management, the course of pain relief follows what you would get with an active drug. The peak relief comes about an hour after it's administered, as it does with the real drug[3]. Hence, in scientific research the placebo effect must be controlled for if the results are to be attributed to the product.

7. **What are the long term effects of the product?** You might be interested in a weight loss drug that definitely works, but if people are dying from the drug, you need to ask yourself if looking slimmer in your **coffin is really what you want.**

A glaring example of this occurred recently when Redux and Phen/fen were pulled from the market. We were told that these drugs were the beginning of the end of obesity with only one serious side effect—primary pulmonary hypertension. Creators of these drugs convinced us that they were innocuous. They simply increase the time serotonin ( a natural brain chemical) remains between brain cells (producing a feeling of being full). Addition of these serotonin uptake inhibitors in pill form simply could not be harmful. But harmful they are— even life threatening. We are now told that one third of the persons taking these drugs have heart valve problems. No matter whom you blame for this scandal, the drug companies, the FDA, the physicians prescribing the drugs, or the individuals taking them, the fact remains that we live in a world where we as consumers must be educated consumers. We can no longer rely on our system to protect our health.

8. **What do other researchers have to say?** If the claims are based on a single study, the advice from experts is to wait for several reliable universities to reproduce the results. The results of such studies should be compared to results conducted by other researchers from reputable institutions. If the claims are based on a single study, the advice from experts is to wait for several reliable universitiesto reproduce the results. Even when the research is well

designed, duplicated, and safety issues have been answered, the results may not be applicable to you. Were the subjects men or women; were they athletes, or sedentary individuals; were they healthy individuals, or individuals with diseases such as diabetes, cancer, or HIV? If you are different from the experimental group, then you should not assume that the results will apply to you.

Here are suggestions published by the FDA. Fraudulent products can often be identified by the types of claims:

1. Claims that the product is a secret cure and use terms such as breakthrough, magical, miracle cure, and new discovery.

2. Pseudomedical jargon such as detoxify, purify, and energize to describe a product's effects. These claims are vague and hard to measure. They make it easier for success to be claimed even though nothing has been accomplished.

3. Claims that the product can cure a wide range of unrelated diseases. No product can do that.

4. Claims that the product is backed by scientific studies, but with no list of references or references that are inadequate. For instance, if a list of references is provided, the citations cannot be traced, or if they are traceable, they are out of date, irrelevant, or poorly designed.

5. Claims that the supplement has only benefits-no side effects. **A product potent enough to help people will be potent enough to cause side effects.**

6. Accusations that the medical profession, drug companies, and the government are suppressing information about a particular treatment. It would be illogical for large numbers of people to withhold information about potential medical therapies when they and their families might benefit from them.

7. Products that claim to be patented to provide health benefits.

REMEMBER: The human body must remain in homeostasis to survive. Homeostasis is the maintenance of constant internal conditions. The body responds to perturbations in internal conditions through corrective responses; if left unopposed, these perturbations would cause unacceptably large changes in internal conditions thereby producing disease or death. Hence, if you overdose on one chemical, the body must rebound by utilizing or producing another chemical that will return the internal conditions to homeostasis. Hence, something so simple as increasing the time serotonin - a natural brain chemical - remains between brain cells forces the body to respond in a way that was totally unforeseen by scientists.

ADVICE: BE CAREFUL WHEN CONTEMPLATING INGESTING ANY NEW PRODUCT ON THE MARKET - THE LIFE YOU SAVE MAY VERY WELL BE YOUR OWN!

# Obstacles to Success

"As you progress through your steps to control, you may encounter certain situations, events, or people that just seem to make it more difficult for you to stick to your program. Before we look at specifics let me remind you that you are in charge - you are the only one who can make change for yourself, who can live a healthier life and can gain control. Do not let anyone or anything get in your way. Develop a strategy - plan ahead and you can overcome any obstacle."

# Friendly Saboteurs

Saboteurs are essentially people who target your behavior for their business. They offer food when it is not wanted, advice whether it is wise or not, and commentary not generally designed to facilitate attainment of goals.

Saboteurs come in so many forms that it is often difficult to spot them until after the fact. Some mean well but produce harm through their ignorance, others are deliberately trying to sabotage, and still others are simply selfish. The only commonality is that regardless of motives, saboteurs try to alter behavior from what should be done to what they want done.

There are several steps in gaining the upper hand over people's efforts to control. The first step is to really convince yourself that you have the right to say "no." The second is to identify the principal saboteurs; they are not always obvious. The next step is to master strategies to produce assertiveness in yourself.

# Traveling

Learning to eat when traveling can be traumatic. Making healthy choices when traveling is a process of "trial and error." You need to slowly learn how to make healthy choices when eating out, how to carry healthy snacks with you when traveling, and how to avoid those "social" alcoholic drinks. In the next section on eating out I've provided some helpful hints.

# Eating Out

Eating out can be traumatic for individuals beginning new lifestyle changes. People need to be educated on how to make wise choices when eating out. Yes, people can eat out and still maintain healthy habits. But don't be fooled! It can be a confusing, difficult task. Remember to stay away from cream sauces and fried foods, and don't be fooled by the word "sautéed."

Read the menu carefully. Key words such as creamy, crunchy, or au gratin signify that the food is probably high in fat. Tempura is the Japanese way of saying "deep fried."

Grilled, broiled, poached, and steamed are low-fat ways of cooking, but they are by no means a guarantee that no fat was added. You need to ask if fat was added.

If soup is on the menu, it's your job to ask if the soup was made with milk or cream. If you're ordering pasta, you need to ask if the pasta was tossed with oil before the sauce was added. Always ask for dressings on the side; you'll gain control over how much fat is added to your food.

Many restaurants are now offering low-fat alternatives to their regular menu. Don't be afraid to ask. Ask about portion sizes as well; don't be afraid to request that half the portion be put aside to be taken home.

In an Italian restaurant, order pasta. Ordering an entrée that's largely spaghetti or linguini will more likely keep the fat calories below 30 percent. Chicken marsala usually has oil or butter added; veal parmigiana has approximately 44 grams of fat; cheese ravioli is almost 40 percent fat; lasagna has over 50 grams of fat; and Fettuccini Alfredo has over 90 grams of fat.

In a Chinese restaurant order extra rice; the more rice, the less fat. Ask for "steamed" vegetables, and don't be afraid to order extra servings. Use your fork or chopsticks to lift the food out of the sauce onto your rice and vegetables leaving excess sauce, egg, and nuts behind.

Don't be fooled in a Mexican restaurant. Tortilla chips are 47 percent fat; refried beans are 39 percent fat; cheese nachos are 62 percent fat; and beef and cheese nachos with sour cream are 59 percent fat. Mexican rice is not as low in fat as white rice from a Chinese restaurant, but with 15 percent fat it still is an accept-able choice. Chicken fajitas are also an acceptable choice at 26 percent fat. Some Mexican restaurants, such as Chili's, are now offering lower fat alterna-tives.

Don't think that because alcoholic beverages are not fat calories they must be okay. Alcohol calories, while not fat calories, are turned into fat by the body. So if you decide to have a drink, skip the dessert.

## Quantity and Timing

Eating too little leads to late day hunger and sometimes binge eating. You can't save food for the evening; if you eat too much in the evening and your body cannot use the food, the extra will be stored in the fat cell. A study by Halberg showed that subjects who ate 2000 calories at breakfast lost weight. When the identical meal was moved to an evening meal, four of the six gained weight, and the remaining two lost less than they did previously (Halberg, 1983).

## Problem Foods and Shopping

Everyone has foods they can't resist; problem foods should not be kept in the house. Stock up on snack foods you don't care for the rest of your family. Don't deprive yourself of your favorite foods; develop a strategy and make a plan to indulge once a month or once a week. When shopping always have a list, and never shop when you're hungry. Avoid the tempting food sections; do not fool yourself into buying treats for the kids or your spouse.

## No Time for Food Preparation

Planning is really the key for this one. Keep your shelves and freezer stocked with healthy choices. If you plan meals weekly, do as much of the preparation ahead as you can; for example, freeze meat in slices for stir-fry. Cook extra amounts on weekends. No time for salad preparation? Try the salad bar at the local grocery store.

## A Holiday or Dinner Guest

One of the most awkward situations is being a guest - generally you have no control over what is being served. The most obvious strategy is to load up on vegetables and take small portions of higher fat items. Keep portions small. Never arrive hungry. Avoid adding extra fat such as butter, sour cream, and gravy. If you are at a buffet or cocktail party with food tables, take what you want and then move away from the food. Offer to bring a dish and make it a healthy one that you can enjoy.

# Table 1
# Carbohydrate Foods

|  | Food Amount | Carbs (g) | Total Calories |
|---|---|---|---|
| Fruits |  |  |  |
| Apple | 1 med | 20 | 80 |
| Orange | 1 med | 20 | 80 |
| Banana | 1 med | 25 | 105 |
| Raisins | ¼ cup | 30 | 120 |
| Vegetables |  |  |  |
| Corn, canned | ½ cup | 18 | 80 |
| Winter squash | ½ cup | 15 | 65 |
| Peas | ½ cup | 10 | 60 |
| Carrot | 1 med | 10 | 40 |
| Green Beans | ½ cup | 7 | 30 |
| Broccoli | 1 stalk | 5 | 30 |
| Zucchini | ½ cup | 4 | 20 |
| Bread |  |  |  |
| Submarine roll | 8" long | 60 | 280 |
| Branola wheat bread | 2 slices | 35 | 210 |
| Lender's Bagel | 1 | 30 | 160 |
| Thomas's English | 1 | 25 | 130 |
| Pita pocket | ½ of 8" round | 22 | 120 |
| Matzo | 1 sheet | 28 | 115 |
| Saltines | 6 | 15 | 90 |
| Graham Crackers | 2 squares | 11 | 60 |
| Grains, pasta, starches |  |  |  |
| Baked potato | 1 large | 55 | 240 |
| Baked beans | 1 cup | 50 | 330 |
| Lentils, cooked | 1 cup | 40 | 215 |

# Table 2
## Fats

|  | Saturated | Monounsaturated | Polyunsaturated |
|---|---|---|---|
| **Bad\*** |  |  |  |
| **(Saturated)** |  |  |  |
| Coconut oil | 90 | 10 | - |
| Palm oil | 50 | 30 | 20 |
| Butter | 65 | 30 | 5 |
| Beef fat | 50 | 45 | 5 |
| Chicken fat | 30 | 50 | 20 |
|  |  |  |  |
| Good |  |  |  |
| Monounsaturated |  |  |  |
| Olive oil | 15 | 75 | 10 |
| Canola oil | 5 | 60 | 35 |
|  |  |  |  |
| So/So |  |  |  |
| Peanut oil | 20 | 50 | 30 |
| Soybean oil | 23 | 62 | 15 |

*Margarine and other trans fatty acids are created when vegetable oils are hardened. Trans fatty acids have been associated with high rates of heart disease.

# Table 3
## Proteins

| Item | Serving Size | Protein (g) |
|---|---|---|
| Meat, poultry, fish | 3 oz. cooked | 21 |
| Milk | 8 oz. | 10 |
| Yogurt | 8 oz. | 8 |
| Cottage cheese | 4 oz. | 13 |
| Eggs (whites) | 1 large | 4 |
| Beans, dried peas, lentils | $\frac{1}{2}$ cup cooked | 7 |

# Table 4

## Serving Size

The number of servings recommended for each group of the food pyramid are expressed as ranges. You should eat at least the lowest number of servings from each of the five major food groups. You need them for the vitamins, minerals, carbohydrates, and protein they provide. Try to pick the lowest fat choices from the food groups—fats, oils, and sweets should be used sparingly! Your age, sex, and activity level determine the number of calories and servings you will need each day.

If you eat a larger portion, count it as more than 1 serving. For example, if you eat a dinner portion of spaghetti that may count as 2 to 3 servings of pasta.

The Pyramid was designed for the general population. Special concerns, such as lactose intolerance or diabetes, and special eating habits, such as those of vegetarians, need to be dealt with on an individualized basis.

## What Is One Serving?

### Milk, Yogurt , and Cheese*
- 1 cup of milk or yogurt
- $1^{1}/_{2}$ oz. natural cheese
- 2 oz. process cheese

### Meat, Poultry, Fish, Dry Beans, Eggs, and Nuts
- 2-3 oz. cooked lean meat, poultry or fish
- $^{1}/_{2}$ cup cooked dry beans, 1 egg, or 2 tbsps. peanut butter count as 1 oz. of lean meat

*Beware: Cheese, eggs, and peanut butter also contain large amounts of saturated fats

### Vegetables
- 1 cup raw leafy vegetables
- $^{1}/_{2}$ cup other vegetables, cooked or chopped raw
- $^{3}/_{4}$ cup vegetable juice

### Fruit
- 1 med. apple, banana, orange
- $^{1}/_{2}$ cup chopped, cooked, or canned fruit
- $^{3}/_{4}$ cup fruit juice

### Bread, Cereal, Rice, and Pasta
- 1 slice of bread
- 1 oz. ready-to-eat cereal
- ½ cup cooked cereal, rice, or pasta

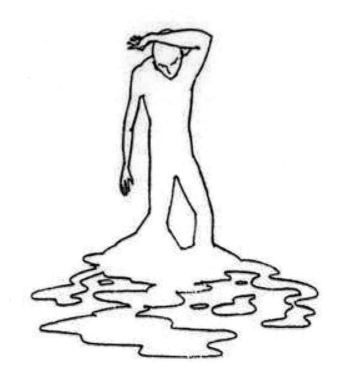

# Chapter 2
# Exercise Basics

# Exercise Basics

No matter what age or ability you are, you need to include exercise in your life. There are three forms that exercise must take for optimum health: cardiorespiratory exercise, muscle strengthening exercise and flexibility exercise (stretching).

Cardiorespiratory exercise consists of continuous large muscle activities that condition the heart, lungs, and circulatory system.

Muscle strengthening exercise consists of resistance exercises that challenge muscles and increase strength.

The benefits of stretching are many and as equally important as cardiorespiratory and muscular fitness. Stretching increases flexibility, coordination, agility and widens the body's freedom of movement. Too little activity causes muscles to shorten and the joint connective tissue (tendons and ligaments) to weaken. When this occurs, ordinary activities of daily life become difficult and painful. Flexibility is directly correlated to functional capacity; i.e., the ability to take care of ourselves.

In order to simplify the task of incorporating exercise into your hectic lifestyle, it is helpful to look at the three phases involved in creating and maintaining an effective exercise program:

1. Getting Started

2. Getting Conditioned

3. Getting Better

# Stage 1 - Getting Started

Many people are overwhelmed by the idea of incorporating regular exercise into their lives. They may have tried to exercise in the past only to get discouraged and give up their programs. Common problems are injuries, lack of time, and boredom. There are some very important steps to take before you embark on your program.

The very first step is to **make the decision** that you are going to become a more active person. You must make a commitment to yourself by making your health a priority - no one can do it for you. Participating in regular physical activity is a way you can take charge of yourself and your health.

The next step is to check with your physician, if necessary. If you are a man over 40 years of age, a woman over 50, or a person with either a chronic disease or risk factors for chronic disease, you need to consult your physician about initiating exercise.

The real secret to a successful exercise program is progression. No matter what age or ability you are you cannot jump off the couch and into a marathon - you need to start with small steps. Remember, the Getting Started phase is for those of you who have not been exercising at all or who have only sporadically exercised. There is no time limit put on this phase - it will be different for everyone.

The most important outcome in this stage is that you will become a regular exerciser and understand the framework of an effective exercise program. Do not progress to phase 2 until you view yourself as an exerciser (for life).

## Cardiorespiratory

Walking is one of the easiest activities for most people to include. Start your program by walking up to 5 minutes each day. Put on a pair of shoes with good support (preferably an athletic shoe) and start to walk. At this point you do not have to worry about how fast or how far you go, you just need to keep moving at an even pace for 5 minutes. This can be done inside or outside.

Depending on your starting point you may continue with this program for several weeks. Be aware of the distance you can cover in 5 minutes. You should notice that you can go farther as your program progresses.

The next step would be extending the cardiorespiratory time from 5 minutes to 10 minutes of continuous activity. The final part of the Getting Started phase is increasing the cardiorespiratory exercise time from 10 minutes to 20 minutes. Initially this can be done by doing two to 10 minute sessions each day.

# Muscle Strengthening

Muscle strengthening exercises should be done with a day of rest between exercises for each specific muscle group; i.e., do dumbbell bentover row every other day, not every day. Try to do at least 8 repetitions of each exercise during the first week. As you feel stronger you can progress to 12 repetitions. When you can do 12 repetitions, add another set of each exercise. During your first week of exercise do each exercise without added resistance in order to learn how to do the motion properly. When you feel comfortable with the movements you can progress to adding resistance. A pair of old panty hose can work like an exercise band for those who need to start with very light resistance. Others may progress to hand weights.

Four Basic exercises in the Getting Started phase include:

1. Supported dumbbell bentover row

2. Leg extension

3. Leg curl

4. Push-ups

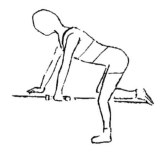 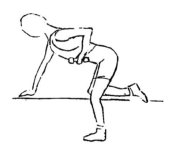

## 1. Supported Dumbbell Bentover row

Bend at the waist with back parallel to the floor. Grasp a dumbell with one hand, and place the other hand and knee on a bench for back support. Pull the dumbell to the chest as you exhale, pause momentarily. Lower slowly (as you inhale) to elbow extended position.

## 2. Leg extension

Put on your ankle weights. Sit back in your chair, roll up the towel and place it under your knees. Gently grasp the chair seat, extend (straighten) one leg horizontally, hold for count of 2, then lower slowly. When your leg is in the straightened position, do not lock your knee. Repeat for several repetitions and then switch to the other leg.

## 3. Leg Curl

With ankle weights on, stand close to the chair holding on to the back. Without moving your upper leg, bend your knee in order to raise the lower leg to the back of the thigh, hold for a count of 2, then slowly lower. Repeat for several repetitions and switch to the other leg.

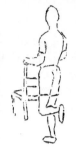

## 4. Push Up

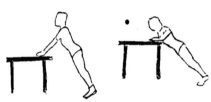

Beginner: Stand about 3 feet away from a counter, or well secured table and place your hands a little more than shoulder width apart, with arms straight. Keeping body straight, bend your arms and slowly lower your chest toward the edge of the counter or table. Then push up to return to the starting position.

Intermediate: Begin on the floor with the hands slightly wider than shoulder width apart and the knees and lower legs on the floor. Lower your straight body until the chest contacts the floor. Press a straight body to full arms extension to return to the starting position.

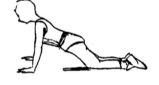

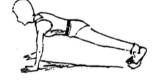

Expert: Begin on the floor with the hands slightly wider than shoulder width apart and the body fully extended (support your body on your hands and toes). Lower your straight body until the chest contacts the floor. Press a straight body to full arms extension to return to the starting position.

## Flexibility

Stretching should be done daily. Specific stretches for upper and lower body will not be described here; however you want to stretch every muscle group, beginning with your neck and progressing to your toes. Never do stretching if you are not warmed up - 5 minutes of walking is perfect.

# Stage 2 - Getting Conditioned

This stage is defined by the American College of Sports Medicine (ACSM), the Centers for Disease Control (CDC), and the Surgeon General as the stage of fitness which will reduce the incidence of all forms of chronic diseases. *So your goal in this stage is to work towards achieving the following guidelines for all three forms of exercise.*

According to the guidelines published by ACSM, CDC, and the Surgeon General, every adult should accumulate 60 minutes or more of moderate-intensity physical activity on most days of the week. The 60 minutes can be accumulated in short bouts of exercise, or 60 minutes in one bout. There is a clear association between total daily or weekly caloric expenditure and cardiovascular disease mortality.

The ACSM guidelines indicate that muscle strengthening exercises should be completed for every large muscle group. These exercises should be performed a minimum of 2 times per week with 8 to 12 repetitions which will produce fatigue of the muscle group. In other words, when you have completed the exercise for a specific muscle group, you simply can not do another exercise because the muscle is fatigued. It is critical to complete muscle strengthening exercises properly and slowly. **Several sessions with a personal trainer at this point would be very advantageous.** A personal trainer should no longer be viewed as a luxury, but as an essential component to your exercise regimen.

The benefits of stretching are many and are equally as important as cardiorespiratory exercise and muscle strengthening exercise. Stretching increases flexibility, coordination, and agility and widens the body's freedom of movement. Too little activity causes muscles to shorten and the joint connective tissue to weaken. When this occurs, ordinary activities of daily life become difficult and painful. Flexibility is directly correlated to functional capacity; i.e., the ability to take care of yourself. ACSM guidelines indicate that exercises should concentrate on slow, easy, movements concentrating on proper form. The stretching regimen should range from ten to fifteen minutes each day, being sure to include all large muscle groups.

These guidelines indicate that all persons should exercise, no matter what age or what limitations exist. Persons with arthritis and joint limitations are specifically mentioned in the guidelines. Exercise is especially critical for these populations. Exercise has been shown to reduce joint pain, increase mobility and independence. Again it doesn't matter how long it takes you to accomplish these goals. The most important outcome in this stage is to become conditioned.

# Stage 3 - Getting Better

Cngratulations for getting to stage 3. You have achieved a level of fitness that will add years to your life. Now the question becomes how do I continue?

This is a great time to look at ways to keep your exercise program challenging and fun. Working with a personal trainer can be very beneficial for your health at this stage, and should no longer be perceived as a luxury for the affluent, or privileged. A qualified personal trainer should be a component of improving your exercise program.

The following are suggestions of some of the ways you can keep your program challenging:

1. Increase your exercise intensity—work harder, not necessarily longer. For example, if you are walking, jogging, or cycling you can add hills to your course.

2. Increase the intensity of your strength workout. Rather than increasing the amount of times you exercise, make the workout harder. Such techniques as slow training, breakdown training, and superset training can be used to increase the intensity (see your trainer for explanations).

3. Try interval training; a method in which you alternate between higher intensity and your regular pace. For example, walking at your usual pace for a few minutes and then jogging for a few minutes.

4. Do some cross training. Incorporate different cardiorespiratory activities. If you spend 30 minutes on cardiorespiratory exercise, you could do 15 minutes of walking and 15 minutes of cycling.

5. Try a competition or sign up for a walk for your favorite cause.

6. Experiment with new activities. There are so many exciting options to put pizzazz in your program, such as hiking, rollerblading, cross country skiing, dancing, or exercise classes.

No matter what you choose to do, the most important thing is to stay active and enjoy what you do!

Visit www.aasdn.org for a list of personal trainers in your area who are also qualified Nutrition Specialists. They can design an exercise program in conjunction with a specialized nutrition program.

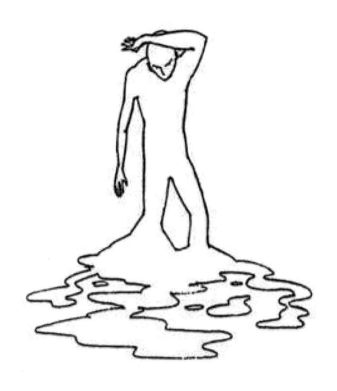

# Part IV
# Menu Planning
# for a
# Healthy Lifestyle

# Energy Intake

The goals of this chapter are to help you determine a range of adequate energy intake (protein, fat, and carbs) and to assist you in menu planning. In determining your range of energy intake, the focus is not to have you count calories, but to learn a pattern of healthy eating. It is more important to concentrate on obtaining adequate amounts of proteins and carbs and limiting fats. Yes, total calories do count, but an extra bagel here and there can be stored in muscle (especially if you have lots of muscle). A donut will be stored in the fat cell! So what kind of calories you consume is just as important as how many calories you consume and when they are eaten.

# Crucial To Your Success

The amount of calories, carbs, proteins, and fat that meet your energy needs will allow you to lose fat without muscle loss if you: (1) Keep the fat grams to the amount allowed, (2) Incorporate the protein grams recommended, (3) Exercise (both cardiovascular and muscle strengthening) a minimum of three times per week, (4) Include lots of fruits and vegetables in your daily menu plan, and (5) Drink six to eight glasses of water per day.

# Step One: Determine Your Energy Intake

Determine your weight and percent body fat. It is essential to know your percent body fat to determine what your daily caloric intake should be; the higher your percent of body fat, the fewer calories your body will utilize. Turn to Table 5 if you are a female or Table 6 if you are a male to determine your range of caloric intake.

# Step Two: Go For It!

Once you have determined your energy intake, turn to the appropriate menu plan designed for your caloric intake to begin your healthy eating program.

Example

Susan is a 45-year old woman who exercises three times a week. She has 35 percent body fat and weighs 130 pounds.

Step 1. From Table 5, Susan determined her caloric needs to be 1900 calories. She should maintain caloric intake at 1800 calories per day to fuel her muscles and to burn fat. Since dieting does not fuel muscles and results in loss of lean body muscle, Susan should not eat less than 1800 calories per day. To be successful in weight loss, she must minimize the fats in her diet and follow the 1800 calorie menu plan.

Step 2. From the 1800 Calorie Menu Plan, Susan will choose one food from each of the three columns at each meal; half the amount of one food from column 2 and one food from column 3 for a morning snack; half the amount of one food from column 2 and one food from column 3 for an afternoon snack; and one food from column 3 for a bedtime snack.

Step 3. Using the 1800 Calorie Menu Plan, Susan will plan each meal incorporating a food from column 1, column 2, and column 3 and will plan her snacks as described above. A sample 1800 calorie menu plan is provided. Susan can also use the sheets provided in the Appendix to track her daily intake.

Step 4. Using the recipes in Part IV, Susan can simply refer to the nutritional information provided for every recipe. For example: if the recipe includes a food from column one and a food from column 2, then all that Susan has to do is add a food from column 3.

## Please Note

Cardiovascular exercise for both men and women should be at such an intensity that perspiration occurs and speech is intermittent.

# Table 5

## For Women Only

Sedentary = Less than three hours/week cardiovascular exercise
Active = Three hours or more/week cardiovascular exercise

| Weight | % Body Fat | Sedentary | Active |
|---|---|---|---|
| 120 | 15-25 | 1800-1750 | 2100-2000 |
| | 26-35 | 1750-1600 | 1900-1800 |
| | >35 | 1500 | 1600 |
| 130 | 15-25 | 1900-1850 | 2100-2000 |
| | 26-35 | 1850-1700 | 2000-1900 |
| | > 35 | 1600 | 1800 |
| 140 | 15-25 | 2000-1900 | 2200-2100 |
| | 26-35 | 1900-1800 | 2100-2000 |
| | > 35 | 1700 | 1900 |
| 150 | 15-25 | 2100-2000 | 2400-2300 |
| | 26-35 | 2000-1900 | 2300-2200 |
| | > 35 | 1750 | 2000 |
| 160 | 15-25 | 2200-2100 | 2600-2400 |
| | 26-35 | 2000-1900 | 2400-2300 |
| | > 35 | 1800 | 2100 |
| 170 | 15-25 | 2300-2200 | 2800-2700 |
| | 26-35 | 2200-2100 | 2700-2600 |
| | > 35 | 1850 | 2200 |
| 180 | 15-25 | 2400-2300 | 3000-2900 |
| | 26-35 | 2300-2100 | 2900-2700 |
| | > 35 | 1900 | 2300 |
| 190 | 15-25 | 2500-2400 | 3200-3100 |
| | 26-35 | 2400-2200 | 3100-2800 |
| | > 35 | 2000 | 2400 |
| 200 | 15-25 | 2800-2700 | 3400-3200 |
| | 26-35 | 2600-2400 | 3200-2900 |
| | > 35 | 2100 | 2600 |
| 201-225 | If you weigh more than 200 | 2200 | 2400 |
| 226-250 | pounds and are above average in | 2300 | 2500 |
| >251 | body fat, use these guidelines. | 2400 | 2600 |

Note: This table is intended to provide an estimate of caloric needs. It is not as accurate as completing the Total Energy Expenditure calculation.

# Table 5
## For Men Only

Sedentary = Less than three hours/week cardiovascular exercise
Active = Three hours or more/week cardiovascular exercise

| Weight | % Body Fat | Sedentary | Active |
|--------|-----------|-----------|--------|
| 140 | 10-19 | 2400-2200 | 2800-2600 |
| | 20-29 | 2200-2000 | 2600-2400 |
| | > 29 | 1800 | 2100 |
| 150 | 10-19 | 2500-2300 | 2900-2700 |
| | 20-29 | 2300-2100 | 2700-2500 |
| | > 29 | 2000 | 2300 |
| 160 | 10-19 | 2700-2500 | 3100-2900 |
| | 20-29 | 2500-2300 | 2900-2700 |
| | > 29 | 2100 | 2500 |
| 170 | 10-19 | 2900-2700 | 3300-3000 |
| | 20-29 | 2700-2500 | 3000-2900 |
| | > 29 | 2300 | 2600 |
| 180 | 10-19 | 3000-2800 | 3400-3200 |
| | 20-29 | 2800-2600 | 3200-3000 |
| | > 29 | 2400 | 2700 |
| 190 | 10-19 | 3200-3000 | 3600-3400 |
| | 20-29 | 3000-2800 | 3400-3200 |
| | > 29 | 2600 | 2800 |
| 200 | 10-19 | 3300-3100 | 3800-3600 |
| | 20-29 | 3100-2900 | 3600-3400 |
| | > 29 | 2700 | 3200 |
| 210 | 10-19 | 3400-3200 | 4000-3800 |
| | 20-29 | 3200-3000 | 3800-3600 |
| | > 29 | 2800 | 3400 |
| 220 | 10-19 | 3600-3400 | 4200-4000 |
| | 20-29 | 3400-3200 | 4000-3800 |
| | > 29 | 2900 | 3600 |
| 230 | 10-19 | 3800-3600 | 4400-4200 |
| | 20-29 | 3600-3400 | 4200-4000 |
| | > 29 | 3100 | 3800 |
| 240 | 10-19 | 4000-3800 | 4600-4400 |
| | 20-29 | 3800-3600 | 4400-4200 |
| | > 29 | 3200 | 4000 |
| 250 | 10-19 | 4200-4000 | 4800-4600 |
| | 20-29 | 4000-3800 | 4600-4400 |
| | >29 | 3300 | 4200 |
| 251-275 | If you weigh more than 250 | 3300 | 3600 |
| 276-300 | pounds and are above average in | 3400 | 3800 |
| > 300 | body fat, use these guidelines. | 3500 | 4000 |

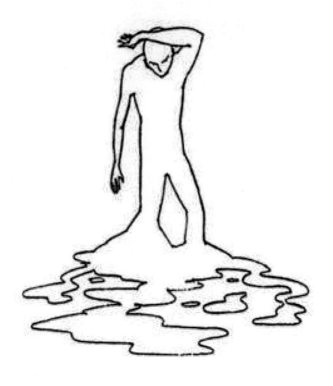

# Menu Plans

The following pages contain menu plans. These plans are designed to teach you healthy patterns of eating. You will notice that not all foods are contained in the columns.

Column 1 contains complex carbohydrates. While the foods are similar in calories, they are not all similar in vitamins and minerals. Try to choose whole grain foods. Remember, the closer to the natural food the better.

Column 2 contains protein foods, while column 3 contains fruits and vegetables which are packed with vitamins and minerals. **You do not have to eat your vegetables cooked** - I use cooked here simply to emphasize portion size. Two cups of a cooked vegetable provide you with 4 servings. You will need to eat double the amount if uncooked (four cups would equal 4 servings). Also, please note that the list is simply a sample list - green beans, turnip greens, etc. would also belong in this list. Juice is listed as a fruit; however, juice does not contain fiber and contains large amounts of sugar. So limit juice to one serving per day.

You will notice there is no column for fats. The menu plans include enough calories to add healthy fats. Be sure to read the Menu Notes to learn how to include these good fats in your menu plan (sample plans are listed for every calorie menu plan).

# 1800 to 2000 Calorie Menu Plan

| | | **Column 1** |
|---|---|---|
| Meals: | Choose one food from each column at each meal. | **Carbohydrates** |
| A.M. Snack: | Choose half the amount of one food choice from column 2 and one food from column 3. | 1 medium bagel (1/2 of a bagel shop bagel) |
| P.M. Snack: | Choose half the amount of one food choice from column 2 and one food from column 3. | 2 servings cereal<br>1½ english muffins |
| Evening Snack: | Choose one food from column 3. | 3 pancakes or (2 pancakes w/2 tbsp. syrup) |

**For 1800** calorie menu follow the above plan.

**For 2000** calorie menu simply change A.M. snack to one food from column 1, half the amount of one food choice from column 2 and one food from column 3.

oatmeal (½ cup uncooked)

2 slices whole grain bread

1 pita bread (2 ounces)

4 med. pretzels (2" each)

4 cups popcorn

---

| **See Sample Menu Plan on how to add essential fats.** |
|---|

**Cooked Foods**

1 medium potato

1 sweet potato

| Note: | Be sure to include variety in your choices. Do not eat four bagels a day or four bananas a day. |
|---|---|

1 cup of one of the following

pasta

corn

peas

winter squash

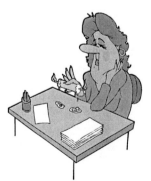

*Remember, stress is perceived.*

## 1800 - 2000 Calorie Menu Plan

| Column 2 | Column 3 |
|---|---|
| **Protein** | **Fruit & Vegetables** |
| 2-8oz oz glasses skim milk | 4 oz. juice |
| $^3/_4$ cup non fat cottage cheese | $^1/_2$ grapefruit |
| 5 egg whites | $^1/_4$ cup pineapple |
| 3 oz. cooked turkey (no skin) | 1 apple |
| 3 oz. tuna (or other white fish) | $^1/_2$ cup grapes or berries |
| 3 oz. cooked chicken(no skin) | 1 small banana |
| 1 scoop of egg white protein supplement (24 g protein) | 1 cup melon |
| 2 cups non-fat yogurt | 1 orange |
| 1 scoop soy protein (24g protein) | $^1/_4$ cup raisins |
| 3 oz. cooked clams, scallops, or shrimp | 4 halves dried apricots |
| | **Cooked Vegetables** |
| | 2 cups carrots |
| | 2 cups broccoli or cauliflower |
| | 2 cups summer squash |
| | 2 cups of asparagus or spinach |
| | 2 cups green or wax beans |

# Menu Notes:

Vegetarian dishes: 1 cup of rice and 1 cup of cooked lentils = 1 food from Column 1 and 1 food from Column 2

At least one choice from Column 3 should be from the vegetable list.

Fats: Notice there is no column for fats. This plan includes enough calories to incorporate approximately 40 to 50 grams of fat. See sample menu plan for hints on how to incorporate these fats.

# 1800 - 2000 Calorie Menu Plan Notes

Fats are essential nutrients. Be sure to add foods listed under Menu Notes in your menu plan. Adding full fat mayonnaise or butter will be adding too many calories (and saturated fats). This menu plan works when you have become accustomed to not adding the full fat versions of these foods. If you add one tablespoon of regular mayonnaise, or one tablespoon of butter you must reduce a food from column 1 by one half, thereby eliminating valuable carbohydrates. Also, the butter or mayonnaise you added will be delivered to your fat cells and will clog your arteries on the way. So begin to decrease these foods and eventually eliminate them from your diet. Always choose low-fat or no-fat alternatives for dairy products.


Remember: Make small changes. Your tastes will change slowly. Too many changes too soon will feel like a diet. Continuously ask yourself if the changes are "lifestyle"; i.e., will you be able to follow this menu plan, on most days, for the rest of your life!

| | |
|---|---|
| Condiments: | You may add small amounts of jelly to your breakfast breads. |
| Soups: | Soups vary widely in caloric and essential nutrients. You can make the following assumptions for the listed soups:<br>1 cup Vegetarian Vegetable (with added vegetables)<br>1/2 food from column 1 & ½ a food from column 3. |
| Cholesterol: | If you have high cholesterol, please read the section "About Cholesterol." |
| Beef: | Beef, pork, and lamb have higher amounts of saturated fats and should be eaten "sparingly". |
| Fats: | Again, as mentioned in your menu plan, be sure to add essential fats in the form of oils and seeds/nuts (be aware of portion sizes).<br>*1 tablespoons of oil (olive, canola, flax, sesame) = 15 g  fat*<br>*2 tblsp nuts/seeds (flax, sesame, sunflower, walnut)  = 10 g fat*<br><br>*1/2 cup soybeans = 5 grams fat    3 ounces cooked salmon = 8 grams fat* |

# 1800 - 2000 Calorie Meal Plan
## Sample Menu Plans

| | **1800** | **2000** |
|---|---|---|
| **Breakfast** | ½ cup uncooked oatmeal<br>8 oz. milk (skim or 1%)<br>8 oz. non-fat yogurt<br>½ grapefruit | ½ cup uncooked oatmeal<br>8 oz. milk (skim or 1%)<br>8 oz. non-fat yogurt<br>½ grapefruit |
| **A.M. Snack** | 8 oz. milk<br>fruit<br>1 T seeds or nuts | 8 oz. milk<br>fruit<br>bagel<br>1 T seeds or nuts |
| **Lunch** | Turkey sandwich with<br>mustard (3 oz. turkey)<br>Salad with 1T oil | Turkey sandwich with<br>mustard (3 oz. turkey)<br>Salad with 1 T oil |
| **P.M. Snack** | 8 oz. milk and fruit<br>or 1 cup yogurt and fruit | 8 oz. milk and fruit<br>or 1 cup yogurt and fruit |
| **Dinner** | 1 cup rice<br>3 oz. salmon<br>2 cups broccoli | 1 cup rice<br>3 oz. salmon<br>2 cups broccoli |
| **Evening Snack** | Fruit<br>1 T seeds or nuts | Fruit<br>1 T seeds or nuts |

# 2200 - 2400 Calorie Menu Plan

| | |
|---|---|
| Meals: | Choose one food from each column at each meal. |
| A.M. Snack: | Choose one food from each column. |
| P.M. Snack: | Choose one food from column 1 and one from column 3. |
| Evening Snack: | Choose one food from column 3. |

**For 2200** calorie menu plan choose snacks as indicated above.

**For 2400** calorie menu plan at evening snack choose 1/2 of the amount of one food from column 1, and 1/2 of the amount of one food from column 2.

---

**See Sample Menu Plan on how to add essential fats.**

---

Note: Be sure to include variety in your choices. Do not eat four bagels a day or four bananas a day.

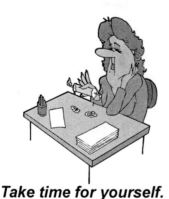

*Take time for yourself.*

## Column 1

### Carbohydrates

1 medium bagel (1/2 of a bagel shop bagel)

2 servings cereal

$1\frac{1}{2}$ english muffins

3 pancakes or
(2 pancakes w/2 tbsp. syrup)

oatmeal ($\frac{1}{2}$ cup uncooked)

2 slices whole grain bread

1 pita bread (2 ounces)

4 med. pretzels (2" each)

4 cups popcorn

**Cooked Foods**

1 medium potato

1 sweet potato

1 cup of one of the following

pasta

corn

peas

winter squash

## 2200 - 2400 Calorie Menu Plan

| Column 2 | Column 3 |
|---|---|
| **Protein** | **Fruit & Vegetables** |
| 2-8oz oz glasses skim milk | 4 oz. juice |
| $^3/_4$ cup non fat cottage cheese | $^1/_2$ grapefruit |
| 5 egg whites | $^1/_4$ cup pineapple |
| 3 oz. cooked turkey (no skin) | 1 apple |
| 3 oz. tuna (or other white fish) | $^1/_2$ cup grapes or berries |
| 3 oz. cooked chicken(no skin) | 1 small banana |
| 1 scoop of egg white protein supplement (24 g protein) | 1 cup melon |
| 2 cups non-fat yogurt | 1 orange |
| 1 scoop soy protein (24g protein) | $^1/_4$ cup raisins |
| 3 oz. cooked clams, scallops, or shrimp | 4 halves dried apricots |
| | **Cooked Vegetables** |
| | 2 cups carrots |
| | 2 cups broccoli or cauliflower |
| | 2 cups summer squash |
| | 2 cups of asparagus or spinach |
| | 2 cups green or wax beans |

# Menu Notes:

Vegetarian dishes: 1 cup of rice and 1 cup of cooked lentils = 1 food from Column 1 and 1 food from Column 2

At least one choice from Column 3 should be from the vegetable list.

Fats: Notice there is no column for fats. This plan includes enough calories to incorporate approximately 49 to 53 grams of fat. See sample menu plan for hints on how to incorporate these fats.

# 2200 - 2400 Calorie Menu Plan Notes

Fats are essential nutrients. Be sure to add foods listed under Menu Notes in your menu plan. Adding full fat mayonnaise or butter will be adding too many calories (and saturated fats). This menu plan works when you have become accustomed to not adding the full fat versions of these foods. If you add one tablespoon of regular mayonnaise, or one tablespoon of butter you must reduce a food from column 1 by one half, thereby eliminating valuable carbohydrates. Also, the butter or mayonnaise you added will be delivered to your fat cells and will clog your arteries on the way. So begin to decrease these foods and eventually eliminate them from your diet. Always choose low-fat or no-fat alternatives for dairy products.

Remember: Make small changes. Your tastes will change slowly. Too many changes too soon will feel like a diet. Continuously ask yourself if the changes are "lifestyle"; i.e., will you be able to follow this menu plan, on most days, for the rest of your life!

| | |
|---|---|
| Condiments: | You may add small amounts of jelly to your breakfast breads. |
| Soups: | Soups vary widely in caloric and essential nutrients. You can make the following assumptions for the listed soups:<br>1 cup Vegetarian Vegetable (with added vegetables)<br>1/2 food from column 1 & ½ a food from column 3. |
| Cholesterol: | If you have high cholesterol, please read the section "About Cholesterol." |
| Beef: | Beef, pork, and lamb have higher amounts of saturated fats and should be eaten "sparingly". |
| Fats: | Again, as mentioned in your menu plan, be sure to add essential fats in the form of oils and seeds/nuts (be aware of portion sizes).<br>*1 tablespoons of oil (olive, canola, flax, sesame) = 15 g fat*<br>*2 tblsp nuts/seeds (flax, sesame, sunflower, walnut) = 10 g fat*<br><br>*1/2 cup soybeans = 5 grams fat    3 ounces cooked salmon = 8 grams fat* |

# 2200-2400 Calorie Meal Plan
## Sample Menu Plans

| | **2200** | **2400** |
|---|---|---|
| **Breakfast** | ½ cup uncooked oatmeal<br>8 oz. milk (skim or 1%)<br>8 oz. non-fat yogurt<br>½ grapefruit | ½ cup uncooked oatmeal<br>8 oz. milk (skim or 1%)<br>8 oz. non-fat yogurt<br>½ grapefruit |
| **A.M. Snack** | 1 bagel<br>¾ cup cottage cheese<br>1 orange<br>1 T nuts or seeds | 1 bagel<br>¾ cup cottage cheese<br>1 orange<br>2 T nuts or seeds |
| **Lunch** | Turkey sandwich with<br>mustard (3 oz. turkey)<br>Salad with 1 T oil | Turkey sandwich with<br>mustard (3 oz. turkey)<br>Salad with 1 T oil |
| **P.M. Snack** | 4 pretzels<br>Fruit | 4 pretzels<br>Fruit |
| **Dinner** | 1 cup rice<br>3 oz. grilled salmon<br>2 cups broccoli<br><br>1 T nuts or seeds | 1 potato w/ no-fat dressing<br>or salsa<br>3 oz. salmon<br>2 cups broccoli<br>1 T nuts or seeds |
| **Evening Snack** | Fruit | 1 serving cereal and<br>8 oz. milk |

## 2600 - 2800 Calorie Menu Plan

| | |
|---|---|
| Meals: | Choose one food from each column at each meal. |
| A.M. Snack: | Choose one food from each column. |
| P.M. Snack: | Choose one food from column 1, half of the amount of one food from column 2, and one food from column 3. |
| Evening Snack: | Choose one food from column 1 and half of the amount of one food from column 2. |

**For 2600** calorie menu plan choose snacks as indicated above.
**For 2800** calorie menu change A.M. Snack to 2 foods from column 1, one food from column 2 and one food from column 3.

**See Sample Menu Plan on how to add essential fats.**

| | |
|---|---|
| Note: | Be sure to include variety in your choices. Do not eat four bagels a day or four bananas a day. |

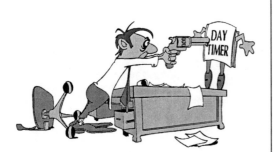

There's got to be a better way to cope!

### Column 1

### Carbohydrates

1 medium bagel (1/2 of a bagel shop bagel)

2 servings cereal

1½ english muffins

3 pancakes or
(2 pancakes w/2 tbsp. syrup)

oatmeal (½ cup uncooked)

2 slices whole grain bread

1 pita bread (2 ounces)

4 med. pretzels (2" each)

4 cups popcorn

### Cooked Foods

1 medium potato

1 sweet potato

1 cup of one of the following

pasta

corn

peas

winter squash

## 2600 - 2800 Calorie Menu Plan

| Column 2 | Column 3 |
|---|---|
| **Protein** | **Fruit & Vegetables** |
| 2-8oz oz glasses skim milk | 4 oz. juice |
| ³/₄ cup non fat cottage cheese | ¹/₂ grapefruit |
| 5 egg whites | ¹/₄ cup pineapple |
| 3 oz. cooked turkey (no skin) | 1 apple |
| 3 oz. tuna (or other white fish) | ¹/₂ cup grapes or berries |
| 3 oz. cooked chicken(no skin) | 1 small banana |
| 1 scoop of egg white protein supplement (24 g protein) | 1 cup melon |
| 2 cups non-fat yogurt | 1 orange |
| 1 scoop soy protein (24g protein) | ¹/₄ cup raisins |
| 3 oz. cooked clams, scallops, or shrimp | 4 halves dried apricots |
| | **Cooked Vegetables** |
| | 2 cups carrots |
| | 2 cups broccoli or cauliflower |
| | 2 cups summer squash |
| | 2 cups of asparagus or spinach |
| | 2 cups green or wax beans |

# Menu Notes:

Vegetarian dishes: 1 cup of rice and 1 cup of cooked lentils = 1 food from Column 1 and 1 food from Column 2

At least one choice from Column 3 should be from the vegetable list.

Fats: Notice there is no column for fats. This plan includes enough calories to incorporate approximately 58 to 62 grams of fat. See sample menu plan for hints on how to incorporate these fats.

# 2600 - 2800 Calorie Menu Plan Notes

Fats are essential nutrients. Be sure to add foods listed under Menu Notes in your menu plan. Adding full fat mayonnaise or butter will be adding too many calories (and saturated fats). This menu plan works when you have become accustomed to not adding the full fat versions of these foods. If you add one tablespoon of regular mayonnaise, or one tablespoon of butter you must reduce a food from column 1 by one half, thereby eliminating valuable carbohydrates. Also, the butter or mayonnaise you added will be delivered to your fat cells and will clog your arteries on the way. So begin to decrease these foods and eventually eliminate them from your diet. Always choose low-fat or no-fat alternatives for dairy products.

Remember: Make small changes. Your tastes will change slowly. Too many changes too soon will feel like a diet. Continuously ask yourself if the changes are "lifestyle"; i.e., will you be able to follow this menu plan, on most days, for the rest of your life!

| | |
|---|---|
| Condiments: | You may add small amounts of jelly to your breakfast breads. |
| Soups: | Soups vary widely in caloric and essential nutrients. You can make the following assumptions for the listed soups: 1 cup Vegetarian Vegetable (with added vegetables) 1/2 food from column 1 & ½ a food from column 3. |
| Cholesterol: | If you have high cholesterol, please read the section "About Cholesterol." |
| Beef: | Beef, pork, and lamb have higher amounts of saturated fats and should be eaten "sparingly". |
| Fats: | Again, as mentioned in your menu plan, be sure to add essential fats in the form of oils and seeds/nuts (be aware of portion sizes). *1 tablespoons of oil (olive, canola, flax, sesame) = 15 g fat* *2 tblsp nuts/seeds (flax, sesame, sunflower, walnut) = 10 g fat* *1/2 cup soybeans = 5 grams fat   3 ounces cooked salmon = 8 grams fat1/2 cup soybeans = 5 grams fat   3 ounces cooked salmon = 8 grams fat* |

# 2600-2800 Calorie Meal Plan
## Sample Menu Plans

|  | **2600** | **2800** |
|---|---|---|
| **Breakfast** | 2 servings cereal (Special K, Total) 8 oz. skim milk 8 oz. non-fat yogurt ½ grapefruit | ½ cup uncooked oatmeal (Special K, Total) 8 oz. skim milk 8 oz. non-fat yogurt ½ grapefruit |
| **A.M. Snack** | 1 pita bread ¾ cup cottage cheese 1 cup melon 1 T nuts or seeds | 2 pita breads ¾ cup cottage cheese 1 cup melon 1 T nuts or seeds |
| **Lunch** | Turkey sandwich with mustard (3-4 oz. turkey) Salad with 1 T oil | Turkey sandwich with mustard (3 oz. turkey) Salad with 1 T oil |
| **P.M. Snack** | 8 oz. skim milk Fruit 4 cups popcorn | 8 oz. skim milk Fruit 4 cups popcorn |
| **Dinner** | 1 potato with no-fat dressing or salsa 3-4 oz. salmon 2 cups carrots Salad with 1 T oil | 1 potato w/ no-fat dressing or salsa 3 oz. salmon 2 cups carrots Salad with 1 T oil |
| **Evening Snack** | 2 serving cereal and 8 oz. milk 1 T nuts or seeds | 2 serving cereal and 8 oz. milk 1 T nuts or seeds |

# 3000 - 3200 Calorie Menu Plan

Meals:

| | |
|---|---|
| Breakfast & Lunch: | For Breakfast and Lunch choose one food plus ½ of a food from each column. |
| Dinner: | Choose one food from each column. |
| A.M. and P.M. Snacks: | Choose one food from column 1, half the amount of one food choice from column 2, and one food from column 3. |
| Evening Snack: | Choose one food from column 1 and one food from column 3. |

**For 3000** calorie menu plan choose snacks as indicated above.
**For 3200** calorie menu plan change A.M. snack to 2 foods from column 1, one half the amount of one food choice from column 2, and one food from column 3.

---

**See Sample Menu Plan on how to add essential fats.**

---

| | |
|---|---|
| Note: | Be sure to include variety in your choices. Do not eat four bagels a day or four bananas a day. |

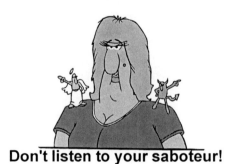

**Don't listen to your saboteur!**

## Column 1

### Carbohydrates

1 medium bagel (1/2 of a bagel shop bagel)

2 servings cereal

1½ english muffins

3 pancakes or
(2 pancakes w/2 tbsp. syrup)

oatmeal (½ cup uncooked)

2 slices whole grain bread

1 pita bread (2 ounces)

4 med. pretzels (2" each)

4 cups popcorn

### Cooked Foods

1 medium potato

1 sweet potato

1 cup of one of the following

pasta

corn

peas

winter squash

# 3000 - 3200 Calorie Menu Plan

| Column 2 | Column 3* |
|---|---|
| **Protein** | **Fruit & Veg** |
| 2-8oz oz glasses skim milk | 4 oz. juice |
| $^3/_4$ cup non fat cottage cheese | $^1/_2$ grapefruit |
| 5 egg whites | $^1/_4$ cup pineapple |
| 3 oz. cooked turkey (no skin) | 1 apple |
| 3 oz. tuna (or other white fish) | $^1/_2$ cup grapes or berries |
| 3 oz. cooked chicken(no skin) | 1 small banana |
| 1 scoop of egg white protein supplement (24 g protein) | 1 cup melon |
| 2 cups non-fat yogurt | 1 orange |
| 1 scoop soy protein (24g protein) | $^1/_4$ cup raisins |
| 3 oz. cooked clams, scallops, or shrimp | 4 halves dried apricots |

**Cooked Vegetables**

2 cups carrots

2 cups broccoli or cauliflower

2 cups summer squash

2 cups asparagus or spinach

# Menu Notes:

Vegetarian dishes: 1 cup of rice and 1 cup of cooked lentils = 1 food from Column 1 and 1 food from Column 2

At least one choice from Column 3 should be from the vegetable list.

Fats: Notice there is no column for fats. This plan includes enough calories to incorporate approximately 66 to 71 grams of fat. See sample menu plan for hints on how to incorporate these fats.

# - 3200 Calorie Menu Plan Notes

are essential nutrients. Be sure to add foods listed under Menu Notes in ur menu plan. Adding full fat mayonnaise or butter will be adding too many calories (and saturated fats). This menu plan works when you have become accustomed to not adding the full fat versions of these foods. If you add one tablespoon of regular mayonnaise, or one tablespoon of butter you must reduce a food from column 1 by one half, thereby eliminating valuable carbohydrates. Also, the butter or mayonnaise you added will be delivered to your fat cells and will clog your arteries on the way. So begin to decrease these foods and eventually eliminate them from your diet. Always choose low-fat or no-fat alternatives for dairy products.

Remember: Make small changes. Your tastes will change slowly. Too many changes too soon will feel like a diet. Continuously ask yourself if the changes are "lifestyle"; i.e., will you be able to follow this menu plan, on most days, for the rest of your life!

Condiments: You may add small amounts of jelly to your breakfast breads.

Soups: Soups vary widely in caloric and essential nutrients. You can make the following assumptions for the listed soups:

1 cup Vegetarian Vegetable (with added vegetables)

1/2 food from column 1 & ½ a food from column 3.

Cholesterol: If you have high cholesterol, please read the section "About Cholesterol."

Beef: Beef, pork, and lamb have higher amounts of saturated fats and should be eaten "sparingly".

Fats: Again, as mentioned in your menu plan, be sure to add essential fats in the form of oils and seeds/nuts (be aware of portion sizes).

*1 tablespoons of oil (olive, canola, flax, sesame) = 15 g fat*

*2 tblsp nuts/seeds (flax, sesame, sunflower, walnut) = 10 g fat*

*1/2 cup soybeans = 5 grams fat    3 ounces cooked salmon = 8 grams fat*

# 3000-3200 Calorie Meal Plan

## Sample Menu Plans

<table>
<tr><th></th><th>3000</th><th>3200</th></tr>
<tr><td>Breakfast</td><td>6 oz. juice (1 1/2 fruits)<br>1/2 bagel with jelly<br>1/2 cup uncooked oatmeal<br>8 oz. skim milk with<br>with egg white protein</td><td>6 oz. juice (1 1/2 fruits)<br>1/2 bagel with jelly<br>1/2 cup uncooked oatmeal<br>8 oz. milk (skim or 1%)<br>with egg white protein</td></tr>
<tr><td>A.M. Snack</td><td>8 oz yogurt<br>Fruit<br>3 pancakes<br>2 T flax seed</td><td>8 oz yogurt<br>Fruit<br>6 pancakes<br>2 T flax seed</td></tr>
<tr><td>Lunch</td><td>Bowl of veg. soup<br>Tuna Sandwich w/tbsp.<br>of low-fat mayo<br>8 oz. milk<br>Large Salad<br>1 T oil</td><td>Bowl of veg. soup<br>Tuna Sandwich w/tbsp.<br>of low-fat mayo<br>8 oz. milk<br>Large Salad<br>1 T oil</td></tr>
<tr><td>P.M. Snack</td><td>2 serving cereal and<br>8 oz. milk<br>Fruit<br>1 T flax seed</td><td>2 serving cereal and<br>8 oz. milk<br>Fruit<br>1 T flax seed</td></tr>
<tr><td>Dinner</td><td>3 oz. salmon<br>1 potato<br>1 cup carrots<br>1 cup broccoli</td><td>3 oz. salmon<br>1 potato<br>1 cup carrots<br>1 cup broccoli</td></tr>
<tr><td>Evening Snack</td><td>4 pretzels<br>Fruit</td><td>4 pretzels<br>Fruit</td></tr>
</table>

# 3400 - 3600 Calorie Menu Plan

| | | Column 1 |
|---|---|---|

**Carbohydrates**

Meals: Choose one food plus 1/2 of a food from each column at each meal.

1 medium bagel (1/2 of a bagel shop bagel)

AM Snack: Choose one food from each column.

2 servings cereal

PM & Evening Snacks: Choose one food from column 1, half the amount of one food choice from column 2, and one food from column 3.

1¹/₂ english muffins

3 pancakes or (2 pancakes w/2 tbsp. syrup)

oatmeal (¹/₂ cup uncooked)

**For 3400** calorie menu plan choose snacks as indicated above.

2 slices whole grain bread

**For 3600** calorie menu plan change A.M. snack to 2 foods from column 1, one food from column 2, and one food from column 3.

1 pita bread (2 ounces)

4 med. pretzels (2" each)

4 cups popcorn

---

**See Sample Menu Plan on how to add essential fats.**

**Cooked Foods**

1 medium potato

Note: Be sure to include a variety in your choices. Do not eat 4 bagels a day or four bananas a day.

1 sweet potato

1 cup of one of the following

pasta

corn

peas

winter squash

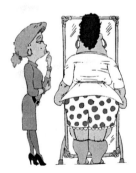

"A journey of a thousand miles begins where one's feet stand."

-Lao Tzu

## 3400 - 3600 Calorie Menu Plan

| Column 2 | Column 3 |
|---|---|
| **Protein** | **Fruit & Vegetables** |
| 2-8oz oz  glasses skim milk | 4 oz. juice |
| $^{3}/_{4}$ cup non fat cottage cheese | $^{1}/_{2}$ grapefruit |
| 5 egg whites | $^{1}/_{4}$ cup pineapple |
| 3 oz. cooked turkey (no skin) | 1 apple |
| 3 oz. tuna (or other white fish) | $^{1}/_{2}$ cup grapes or berries |
| 3 oz. cooked chicken(no skin) | 1 small banana |
| 1 scoop of egg white protein supplement (24 g protein) | 1 cup melon |
| 2 cups non-fat yogurt | 1 orange |
| 1 scoop soy protein (24g protein) | $^{1}/_{4}$ cup raisins |
| 3 oz. cooked clams, scallops, or shrimp | 4 halves dried apricots |

**Cooked Vegetables**

2 cups carrots

2 cups broccoli or cauliflower

2 cups summer squash

2 cups asparagus or spinach

# Menu Notes:

Vegetarian dishes: 1 cup of rice and 1 cup of cooked lentils = 1 food from Column 1 and 1 food from Column 2

At least one choice from Column 3 should be from the vegetable list.

Fats: Notice there is no column for fats. This plan includes enough calories to incorporate approximately 75 to 80 grams of fat. See sample menu plan for hints on how to incorporate these fats.

# 3400 - 3600 Calorie Menu Plan Notes

Fats are essential nutrients. Be sure to add foods listed under Menu Notes in your menu plan. Adding full fat mayonnaise or butter will be adding too many calories (and saturated fats). This menu plan works when you have become accustomed to not adding the full fat versions of these foods. If you add one tablespoon of regular mayonnaise, or one tablespoon of butter you must reduce a food from column 1 by one half, thereby eliminating valuable carbohydrates. Also, the butter or mayonnaise you added will be delivered to your fat cells and will clog your arteries on the way. So begin to decrease these foods and eventually eliminate them from your diet. Always choose low-fat or no-fat alternatives for dairy products.

Remember: Make small changes. Your tastes will change slowly. Too many changes too soon will feel like a diet. Continuously ask yourself if the changes are "lifestyle"; i.e., will you be able to follow this menu plan, on most days, for the rest of your life!

| | |
|---|---|
| Condiments: | You may add small amounts of jelly to your breakfast breads. |
| Soups: | Soups vary widely in caloric and essential nutrients. You can make the following assumptions for the listed soups: |
| | 1 cup Vegetarian Vegetable (with added vegetables) |
| | 1/2 food from column 1 & ½ a food from column 3. |
| Cholesterol: | If you have high cholesterol, please read the section "About Cholesterol." |
| Beef: | Beef, pork, and lamb have higher amounts of saturated fats and should be eaten "sparingly". |
| Fats: | Again, as mentioned in your menu plan, be sure to add essential fats in the form of oils and seeds/nuts (be aware of portion sizes). |

*1 tablespoons of oil (olive, canola, flax, sesame) = 15 g fat*

*2 tblsp nuts/seeds (flax, sesame, sunflower, walnut)  = 10 g fat*

*1/2 cup soybeans = 5 grams fat    3 ounces cooked salmon = 8 grams fat*

# 3400 - 3600 Calorie Meal Plan

## Sample Menu Plans

| | **3400** | **3600** |
|---|---|---|
| **Breakfast** | 6 oz. juice (1 1/2 fruits)<br>3 pancakes (use 3 egg whites)<br>2 tbsp. syrup<br>½ bagel<br>8 oz. milk w/ egg white protein | 6 oz. juice (1 1/2 fruits)<br>3 pancakes (use 3 egg whites)<br>2 tbsp. syrup<br>½ bagel<br>8 oz. milk w/ egg white protein |
| **A.M. Snack** | ½ cup uncooked oatmeal<br>16 oz. milk<br>Fruit<br>2 T flax seed | 1 cup uncooked oatmeal<br>16 oz milk<br>Fruit<br>2 T flax seed |
| **Lunch** | Bowl of veg. soup<br>Tuna sandwich with<br>2 tbsp. low-fat mayo<br>8 oz. milk<br>1 1/2 Fruit servings | Bowl of veg. soup<br>Tuna sandwich with<br>2 tbsp. low-fat mayo<br>8 oz. milk<br>1 1/2 Fruit servings |
| **P.M. Snack** | yogurt<br>4 pretzels<br>Fruit | 1.5 oz. cooked chicken<br>2 slices of bread<br>Fruit |
| **Dinner** | 5-6 oz. salmon<br>1½ potatoes<br>1 cup carrots<br>1 cup broccoli<br>salad<br>1 T oil | 5-6 oz. salmon<br>1½ potatoes<br>1 cup carrots<br>1 cup broccoli<br>salad<br>1 T oil |
| **Evening Snack** | 2 serving cereal<br>8 oz. skim milk<br>Fruit<br>1 T flax seed | 2 serving cereal<br>8 oz. skim milk<br>Fruit<br>1 flax seed |

# 3800 - 4000 Calorie Menu Plan

Meals: Choose one food plus an additonal half of a food from each column at each meal.

A.M. & P.M. Choose two foods from column 1, one food from column 2 and one food from column 3.

Evening Snack: Choose one food from each column.

**For 3800** calorie menu plan choose snacks as indicated above.
**For 4000** calorie menu plan change evening snack to same as A.M. and P.M. snack.

> **See Sample Menu Plan on how to add essential fats.**

Note: Be sure to include variety in your choices. Do not eat four bagels a day or four bananas a day.

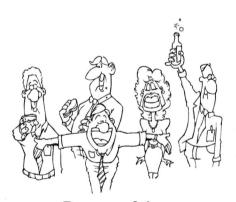

**Beware of the friendly saboteurs!**

## Column 1

### Carbohydrates

1 medium bagel (1/2 of a bagel shop bagel)

2 servings cereal

$1\frac{1}{2}$ english muffins

3 pancakes or (2 pancakes w/2 tbsp. syrup)

oatmeal ($\frac{1}{2}$ cup uncooked)

2 slices whole grain bread

1 pita bread (2 ounces)

4 med. pretzels (2" each)

4 cups popcorn

### Cooked Foods

1 medium potato

1 sweet potato

1 cup of one of the following

pasta

corn

peas

winter squash

# 3800-4000 Calorie Menu Plan

| Column 2 | Column 3 |
|---|---|
| **Protein** | **Fruit & Vegetables** |
| 2-8oz oz glasses skim milk | 4 oz. juice |
| $^3/_4$ cup non fat cottage cheese | $^1/_2$ grapefruit |
| 5 egg whites | $^1/_4$ cup pineapple |
| 3 oz. cooked turkey (no skin) | 1 apple |
| 3 oz. tuna (or other white fish) | $^1/_2$ cup grapes or berries |
| 3 oz. cooked chicken(no skin) | 1 small banana |
| 1 scoop of egg white protein supplement (24 g protein) | 1 cup melon |
| 2 cups non-fat yogurt | 1 orange |
| 1 scoop soy protein (24g protein) | $^1/_4$ cup raisins |
| 3 oz. cooked clams, scallops, or shrimp | 4 halves dried apricots |
| | **Cooked Vegetables** |
| | 2 cups carrots |
| | 2 cups broccoli or cauliflower |
| | 2 cups summer squash |
| | 2 cups asparagus or spinach |

# Menu Notes:

Vegetarian dishes: 1 cup of rice and 1 cup of cooked lentils = 1 food from Column 1 and 1 food from Column 2

At least one choice from Column 3 should be from the vegetable list.

Fats: Notice there is no column for fats. This plan includes enough calories to incorporate approximately 80 to 90 grams of fat. See sample menu plan for hints on how to incorporate these fats.

# 3800 - 4000 Calorie Menu Plan Notes

Fats are essential nutrients. Be sure to add foods listed under Menu Notes in your menu plan. Adding full fat mayonnaise or butter will be adding too many calories (and saturated fats). This menu plan works when you have become accustomed to not adding the full fat versions of these foods. If you add one tablespoon of regular mayonnaise, or one tablespoon of butter you must reduce a food from column 1 by one half, thereby eliminating valuable carbohydrates. Also, the butter or mayonnaise you added will be delivered to your fat cells and will clog your arteries on the way. So begin to decrease these foods and eventually eliminate them from your diet. Always choose low-fat or no-fat alternatives for dairy products.

Remember:  Make small changes.  Your tastes will change slowly.  Too many changes too soon will feel like a diet.  Continuously ask yourself if the changes are "lifestyle"; i.e., will you be able to follow this menu plan, on most days, for the rest of your life!

Condiments:     You may add small amounts of jelly to your breakfast breads.

Soups:          Soups vary widely in caloric and essential nutrients. You can make the following assumptions for the listed soups:

                1 cup Vegetarian Vegetable (with added vegetables)

                1/2 food from column 1 & ½ a food from column 3.

Cholesterol:    If you have high cholesterol, please read the section "About Cholesterol."

Beef:           Beef, pork, and lamb have higher amounts of saturated fats and should be eaten "sparingly".

Fats:           Again, as mentioned in your menu plan, be sure to add essential fats in the form of oils and seeds/nuts (be aware of portion sizes).

                *1 tablespoons of oil (olive, canola, flax, sesame) = 15 g fat*

                *2 tblsp nuts/seeds (flax, sesame, sunflower, walnut) = 10 g fat*

                *1/2 cup soybeans = 5 grams fat    3 ounces cooked salmon = 8 grams fat*

# 3800 - 4000 Calorie Meal Plan
## Sample Menu Plans

|  | **3800** | **4000** |
|---|---|---|
| **Breakfast** | 6 oz. juice (1 1/2 fruits)<br>3 pancakes (use 3 egg whites)<br>2 tbsp. syrup<br>½ bagel<br>8 oz. milk w/ egg white protein | 6 oz. juice (1 1/2 fruits)<br>3 pancakes (use 3 egg whites)<br>2 tbsp. syrup<br>½ bagel<br>8 oz. milk w/ egg white protein |
| **A.M. Snack** | 16 oz milk<br>1 cup oatmeal<br>Fruit<br>2 T flaxseed | 16 oz. milk<br>1 cup oatmeal<br>fruit<br>2 T flaxseed |
| **Lunch** | Bowl of veg. soup<br>Tuna sandwich with<br>2 tbsp. low-fat mayo<br>8 oz. milk<br>1 1/2 Fruit servings | Bowl of veg. soup<br>Tuna sandwich with<br>2 tbsp. low-fat mayo<br>8 oz. milk<br>1 1/2 Fruit servings |
| **P.M. Snack** | 3 oz. cooked chicken<br>2 slices of bread<br>Fruit<br>4 pretzels | 3 oz. cooked chicken<br>2 slices of bread<br>Fruit<br>4 pretzels |
| **Dinner** | 5-6 oz. fish<br>1½ potatoes<br>1 cup carrots<br>1 cup broccoli<br>salad<br>1 T oil | 5-6 oz. fish<br>1½ potatoes<br>1 cup carrots<br>1 cup broccoli<br>salad<br>1 T oil |
| **Evening Snack** | 2 serving cereal<br>16 oz. skim milk<br>Fruit<br>1 T flaxseed | 4 serving cereal<br>16 oz. skim milk<br>Fruit<br>1 T flaxseed |

# 4200 - 4400 Calorie Menu Plan

| | |
|---|---|
| Meals: | Choose 2 foods from each column. |
| A.M. & P.M. | Choose 2 foods from column1, one food from column 2, and 2 foods from column 3. |
| Evening Snack: | Choose one food from each column. |

**For 4200** calorie menu plan choose snacks as indicated above.
**For 4400** calorie menu plan change A.M. snack to three foods from column 1, one food from column 2, and two foods from column 3.

---

**See Sample Menu Plan on how to add essential fats.**

---

| | |
|---|---|
| Note: | Be sure to include variety in your choices. Do not eat four bagels a day or four bananas a day. |

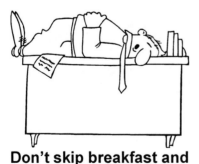

**Don't skip breakfast and lunch!**

## Column 1

### Carbohydrates

1 medium bagel (1/2 of a bagel
    shop bagel)

2 servings cereal

$1^{1}/_{2}$ english muffins

3 pancakes or
(2 pancakes w/2 tbsp. syrup)

oatmeal ($^{1}/_{2}$ cup uncooked)

2 slices whole grain bread

1 pita bread (2 ounces)

4 med. pretzels (2" each)

4 cups popcorn

### Cooked Foods

1 medium potato

1 sweet potato

1 cup of one of the following

pasta

corn

peas

winter squash

## 4200-4400 Calorie Menu Plan

| Column 2 | Column 3 |
|---|---|
| **Protein** | **Fruit & Vegetables** |
| 2-8oz oz glasses skim milk | 4 oz. juice |
| $^3/_4$ cup non fat cottage cheese | $^1/_2$ grapefruit |
| 5 egg whites | $^1/_4$ cup pineapple |
| 3 oz. cooked turkey (no skin) | 1 apple |
| 3 oz. tuna (or other white fish) | $^1/_2$ cup grapes or berries |
| 3 oz. cooked chicken(no skin) | 1 small banana |
| 1 scoop of egg white protein supplement (24 g protein) | 1 cup melon |
| 2 cups non-fat yogurt | 1 orange |
| 1 scoop soy protein (24g protein) | $^1/_4$ cup raisins |
| 3 oz. cooked clams, scallops, or shrimp | 4 halves dried apricots |
| | **Cooked Vegetables** |
| | 2 cups carrots |
| | 2 cups broccoli or cauliflower |
| | 2 cups summer squash |
| | 2 cups asparagus or spinach |

# Menu Notes:

Vegetarian dishes: 1 cup of rice and 1 cup of cooked lentils = 1 food from Column 1 and 1 food from Column 2

At least one choice from Column 3 should be from the vegetable list.

Fats: Notice there is no column for fats. This plan includes enough calories to incorporate approximately 90 to 98 grams of fat. See sample menu plan for hints on how to incorporate these fats.

# 4200 - 4400 Calorie Menu Plan Notes

Fats are essential nutrients. Be sure to add foods listed under Menu Notes in your menu plan. Adding full fat mayonnaise or butter will be adding too many calories (and saturated fats). This menu plan works when you have become accustomed to not adding the full fat versions of these foods. If you add one tablespoon of regular mayonnaise, or one tablespoon of butter you must reduce a food from column 1 by one half, thereby eliminating valuable carbohydrates. Also, the butter or mayonnaise you added will be delivered to your fat cells and will clog your arteries on the way. So begin to decrease these foods and eventually eliminate them from your diet. Always choose low-fat or no-fat alternatives for dairy products.

Remember: Make small changes. Your tastes will change slowly. Too many changes too soon will feel like a diet. Continuously ask yourself if the changes are "lifestyle"; i.e., will you be able to follow this menu plan, on most days, for the rest of your life!

| | |
|---|---|
| Condiments: | You may add small amounts of jelly to your breakfast breads. |
| Soups: | Soups vary widely in caloric and essential nutrients. You can make the following assumptions for the listed soups:<br>1 cup Vegetarian Vegetable (with added vegetables)<br>1/2 food from column 1 & ½ a food from column 3. |
| Cholesterol: | If you have high cholesterol, please read the section "About Cholesterol." |
| Beef: | Beef, pork, and lamb have higher amounts of saturated fats and should be eaten "sparingly". |
| Fats: | Again, as mentioned in your menu plan, be sure to add essential fats in the form of oils and seeds/nuts (be aware of portion sizes).<br>*1 tablespoons of oil (olive, canola, flax, sesame) = 15 g fat*<br>*2 tblsp nuts/seeds (flax, sesame, sunflower, walnut)  = 10 g fat*<br>*1/2 cup soybeans = 5 grams fat    3 ounces cooked salmon = 8 grams fat* |

# 4200-4400 Calorie Meal Plan

## Sample Menu Plans

| | **4200** | **4400** |
|---|---|---|
| **Breakfast** | grapefruit<br>4 pancakes (use 3 egg whites)<br>4 tbsp. syrup<br>16 oz. milk<br>w/ egg white protein<br>2 T flax seed | grapefruit<br>4 pancakes (use 3 egg whites)<br>4 tbsp. syrup<br>16 oz. milk<br>w/ egg white protein<br>2 T flax seed |
| **A.M. Snack** | 2 bagels<br>¾ cup cottage cheese<br>(no-fat or low-fat)<br>2 cups melon | 3 bagels<br>¾ cup cottage cheese<br>(no-fat or low-fat)<br>2 cups melon |
| **Lunch** | Two tuna sandwiches<br>with 2 tbsp. low-fat mayo<br>2 apples | Two tuna sandwiches<br>with 2 Tbsp. low-fat mayo<br>2 apples |
| **P.M. Snack** | salad<br>4 slices bread<br>3 oz. cooked chicken<br>orange<br>1 T oil | 2-4 cups salad w/tbsp.<br>of oil & vinegar<br>1 cup pasta<br>3 oz. cooked chicken |
| **Dinner** | 5-6 oz. salmon<br>2 potatoes<br>2 cups carrots<br>salad<br>1 T oil | 5-6 oz. salmon<br>2 potatoes<br>2 cups carrots<br>salad<br>1 T oil |
| **Evening Snack** | 2 serving cereal<br>16 oz. skim milk<br>Fruit | 2 serving cereal<br>16 oz. skim milk<br>Fruit |

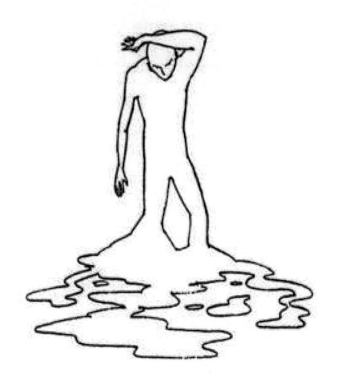

# Part V
# Recipes for Complete Meals

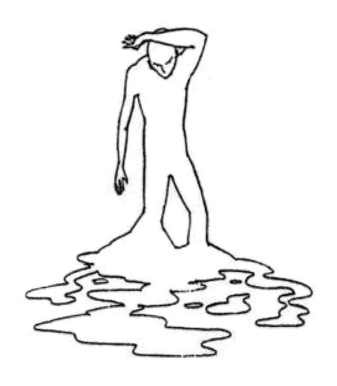

# Chapter 1
# Breakfast
# Healthy Beginnings

# Fruit Smoothie

Breakfast in a glass—high energy fruit drink that gets its sweetness from fruit, not sugar! Fruit adds fiber, vitamins and great taste, not fat. Ideal for breakfast on the run, it takes only 15 minutes to prepare!

## Serves 1

## Ingredients

| | |
|---|---|
| 1 | cup plain nonfat yogurt |
| 1 | cup skim milk |
| ½ | cup fresh strawberries (or unsweetened strawberries, partially thawed) |
| ½ | banana, sliced |
| 1 | tablespoon wheat germ (optional) |
| ½ | teaspoon vanilla extract |
| ¼ | teaspoon ground cinnamon or nutmeg |
| 4 | ice cubes |

Mint sprigs for garnish

## Preparation

- In a blender, combine the yogurt, milk, fruit, wheat germ, vanilla and cinnamon. Add ice cubes.
- Blend until smooth and foamy, about 30 seconds. If mixture is too thick, add a few more ice cubes and blend until smooth.
- Pour mixture into a chilled glass. Garnish with mint sprigs and serve.

## Try This

Don't be afraid to experiment. Substitute your favorite fruits to create delicious blends. Use about 1 cup of fruit. Try using flavored nonfat yogurt.

## Hint

Add a bagel or other food item from Column 1 to make this breakfast complete.

## Per Serving

| | | | |
|---|---|---|---|
| Calories | 260 (2% from fat) | Fat | 5g |
| Carbohydrates | 45g | Protein | 20g |

## Includes

1 food from Column 2 and 2 foods from Column 3

# Cinnamon French Toast

A delicious low-fat treat—made with egg whites to cut cholesterol and with French or Italian bread to lower fat. Serve with reduced-calorie syrup and cinnamon sugar, or for an even lighter meal serve with fresh fruit. Prepare and cook in 20 minutes!

## Serves 4

## Ingredients

| | |
|---|---|
| 1 | large egg |
| 4 | egg whites |
| ¼ | cup skim milk |
| ½ | teaspoon vanilla extract |
| ½ | teaspoon ground cinnamon |
| ⅛ | teaspoon ground nutmeg |
| 8 | 1 inch thick diagonally cut slices French or Italian bread |

Cinnamon sugar and reduced-calorie maple syrup or freshfruit for topping

## Preparation

- In shallow bowl beat the egg and egg whites with wire whisk or fork until foamy. Add milk, vanilla, cinnamon, and nutmeg. Beat well; set aside.
- Preheat oven to 200° F. Spray a large nonstick skillet with light coat of vegetable cooking spray; heat over medium heat.
- Dip 4 of the bread slices into the egg mixture, turning to coat and draining excess back into the dish. Place coated slices on skillet and cook until golden brown, about 1 to 2 minutes per side.
- Transfer cooked slices to a plate; keep warm in oven. Dip remaining slices in egg mixture; cook as directed. Spray skillet with vegetable cooking spray as needed.
- Serve French toast sprinkled lightly with cinnamon sugar and topped with maple syrup or fresh fruit. Serve immediately.

## Hint

Add a glass of milk (8 oz.) and top french toast with fruit to make this breakfast complete.

## Per Serving

| | | | |
|---|---|---|---|
| Calories | 180 (5% from fat) | Fat | 1g |
| Carbohydrates | 31g | Protein | 12g |

## Includes

1 food from Column 1 and ½ food from Column 2

# Strawberry Muffins

Make these tasty low-fat, carbo-packed muffins with fresh berries when in season or with frozen berries. Strawberries are high in Vitamin C and fiber. Takes only 15 minutes to prepare, 20 minutes to bake.

## Makes 12 Muffins

## Ingredients

| | |
|---|---|
| 2$\frac{1}{3}$ | cups all-purpose flour |
| $\frac{3}{4}$ | cup granulated sugar |
| $\frac{1}{4}$ | cup firmly packed light brown sugar |
| 2$\frac{1}{2}$ | teaspoons baking powder |
| $\frac{1}{8}$ | teaspoon salt |
| 1 | cup fresh or thawed frozen strawberries, chopped |
| 1 | cup skim milk and add a pkg of powdered milk (1 quart) |
| $\frac{1}{3}$ | cup non-fat vanilla yogurt |
| 3 | egg whites, lightly beaten |
| 1 | teaspoon vanilla extract |

## Preparation

- Preheat oven to 400° F. Spray a 12-cup muffin pan with vegetable cooking spray or line with paper liners. Set aside.
- In a medium bowl, combine flour, granulated sugar, brown sugar, baking powder, and salt. Mix well. Stir in strawberries.
- In a small bowl, combine milk, yogurt, egg, and vanilla. Mix welland add to dry ingredients. Stir until just combined; do not overmix. Fill each muffin cup about two-thirds full.
- Bake until tops are firm and golden, about 20 minutes. Let cool 5 minutes; remove muffins from pan and cool completely.

## Try This

You can freeze muffins for up to 1 month. Cool completely after baking then tightly foil-wrap muffins individually. To serve, preheat oven to 350° F and heat the foil-wrapped frozen muffin for about 15 minutes.

## Hint

Add 1$\frac{1}{2}$ glasses of milk and a banana to make this breakfast complete.

## Per Muffin

| | | | |
|---|---|---|---|
| Calories | 204 (4% from fat) | Fat | 1g |
| Carbohydrates | 37g | Protein | 15g |

## Includes

1 food from Column 1, 1food from Column 2 and ½ food from Column 3

# Streusel Coffee Cake

This coffee cake is just the thing for weekday breakfasts or afternoon snacks. Nonfat sour cream gives the taste of richness without all the fat; indulge your sweet tooth with a touch of cinnamon. For a twist, add thin slices of fruit over the batter before adding the topping.

## Serves 10 slices

### Ingredients

2¼   cups all-purpose flour
½     cup granulated sugar
1     tablespoon baking powder
1     teaspoon ground cinnamon
6     egg whites
½     cup nonfat sour cream
½     cup skim milk
1     tablespoon canola oil

### Topping

¼     cup all-purpose flour
1     teaspoon ground cinnamon
2     tbls packed light brown sugar
2     tablespoons chilled margarine cut into small pieces

## Preparation

- Preheat oven to 375° F. Spray an 8-inch springform pan with vegetable cooking spray and set aside.
- Prepare topping in a small bowl. Combine dry ingredients. Using a pastry blender or 2 knives, cut in margarine until coarse crumbs form. Set aside.
- Prepare cake using a medium bowl. Combine dry ingredients; mix well. In a large bowl, whisk egg whites, sour cream, milk and oil. Add flour mixture; stir until just combined. Spoon batter into prepared pan.
- Sprinkle topping over batter. Bake until a toothpick inserted in center comes out clean, about 40 minutes. Place pan on a wire rack; cool for 10 minutes. Remove side of pan; cool cake completely.

## Hint

Add a glass of milk and an apple to make this breakfast complete.

## Per Slice

| | | | |
|---|---|---|---|
| Calories | 225 (17% from fat) | Fat | 4g |
| Carbohydrates | 39g | Protein | 8g |

## Includes

1 food from Column 1and ½ food from Column 2

# Cottage Cheese Crepes

Crepes filled with cottage cheese and topped with sweet berries. Cottage cheese provides a good source of calcium and protein, raspberries provide fiber, and a dash of vanilla enhances the flavor of these delicious crepes without adding to the fat.

## Serves 4

## Ingredients

| | |
|---|---|
| 1½ | cups low-fat milk |
| ½ | cup all-purpose flour |
| 2 | large eggs |
| 1 | teaspoon olive oil |
| ¼ | teaspoon vanilla extract |
| ⅛ | teaspoon salt |
| 2 | cups non-fat cottage cheese |
| 2 | cups mixed fresh blueberries, raspberries, and sliced strawberries |

Confectioners' sugar

## Preparation

- Whisk together milk, flour, eggs, oil, vanilla, and salt. Mix well. Chill batter for 30 minutes.
- Spray bottom of a nonstick 8-inch skillet with vegetable cooking spray. Place skillet over medium heat until hot but not smoking. Pour ¼ cup of batter into pan, quickly tilting it in all directions so batter covers bottom. Cook until crepe bottom is golden, about 1 minute. Turn crepe over; cook for 1 minute.
- Transfer crepe to a large plate. Repeat with more cooking spray and remaining batter, stacking and placing a sheet of waxed paper between each crepe.
- Place crepes on individual plates. Spoon cottage cheese evenly on half of each crepe. Fold crepe over filling; fold again to form a triangle. Spoon berries over crepes. Dust with confectioners' sugar. Serve immediately. (Crepes can also be wrapped in foil, each separated by wax paper and frozen for up to 2 months.)

## Hint:

Add a bagel or slice of toast to make this breakfast complete.

## Per Serving

| | | | |
|---|---|---|---|
| Calories | 220 (10% from fat) | Fat | 2g |
| Carbohydrates | 29g | Protein | 22g |

## Includes

½ food from Column 1, 1 food from Column 2 & 1 food from Column 3

# Apple Cran Cakes

Fruit filled pancakes that will make your mouth water—terrific recipe for a fantastic weekend brunch. Just the thing to take the chill off a cool morning. Apples and cranberries add additional fiber. Takes only 10 minutes to prepare and minutes to cook.

## Serves 4

## Ingredients

| | |
|---|---|
| 1½ | cups all-purpose flour |
| 3 | tablespoons granulated sugar |
| 1¾ | teaspoons baking powder |
| 1 | teaspoon ground cinnamon |
| 1 | large egg white, lightly beaten |
| 1 | tablespoon margarine, melted |
| 1 | cup skim milk, and mix 1package (1 quart) powdered milk |
| 1 | Granny Smith apple, peeled and finely chopped (about 1 cup) |
| ½ | cup fresh or frozen, thawed cranberries |

Reduced-calorie maple syrup or all-fruit preserves (optional) for topping

## Preparation

- In a large bowl, sift together flour, sugar, baking powder, and cinnamon. Mix well.
- In a medium bowl, combine egg white, margarine, and milk and mix well. Stir in apple and cranberries.
- Stir fruit mixture into flour mixture until just combined. Batter will be lumpy.
- Heat a large nonstick skillet or griddle over medium heat. Pour batter into skillet making 3-inch rounds; repeat with remaining batter.
- Cook until tops are bubbly, about 2 minutes. Flip pancakes. Cook until golden, 1 minute longer. Cook remaining pancakes as directed. Top with syrup or preserves if desired and serve immediately.

## Hint

This breakfast is complete as is! YEA!

## Per Serving

| | | | |
|---|---|---|---|
| Calories | 365 (7% from fat) | Fat | 3g |
| Carbohydrates | 57g | Protein | 19g |

## Includes

1 food from Column 1, 1food from Column 2 & 1 food from Column 3

# Energy Bars

Here's a high energy bar you can make yourself without all the added sugar. A great choice for either a quick breakfast on the go or a healthy, carbo-loaded snack!

## Serves 6 bars

## Ingredients

1      20 ounce can unsweetened crushed pineapple
1      cup mixed dried fruit pieces
2      cups oats, quick or regular
¼      teaspoon salt (optional)
nonstick cooking spray

## Preparation

- In a food processor with a cutting blade, purée the fruits together. Mix oats and salt in a large bowl. Add the blended fruits; mix well.
- Spray a 9-inch square baking pan with nonstick spray. Add oat and fruit mixture to pan and press in evenly. Bake at 250° F for approximately 2½ hours. Cut into bars after one hour in the oven. Continue baking until firm. Cool and wrap into individual servings. Store in refrigerator or freezer.

## Try This

For variation in flavor, use two cups of any fresh or canned fruit and one cup of any dried fruit. Baking time may vary depending on the type of fruit you use.

## Hint

Add yogurt and fruit to complete breakfast.

## Per Bar

| | | | |
|---|---|---|---|
| Calories | 244 (2% from fat) | Fat | 2g |
| Carbohydrates | 50g | Protein | 8g |

## Includes

1 food from Column 1, ½ food from Column 2 & ½ food from Column 3

# Breakfast Burrito

A quick, easy breakfast with a Mexican flare, this burrito is a great source of protein and is low in fat.

## Serves 1

## Ingredients

| | |
|---|---|
| 4 | egg whites |
| 1 | whole egg |
| 1 | tortilla shell |
| 1 | teaspoon grated cheese |

salsa

## Preparation

- Scramble four egg whites and one whole egg in non-stick pan.
- Place on awarm tortilla shell, add teaspoon grated cheese and roll up.
- Top with salsa.

## Hint

Top this breakfast off with a fruit to make it complete.

## Per Serving

| | | | |
|---|---|---|---|
| Calories | 368 (15% from fat) | Fat | 6g |
| Carbohydrates | 55g | Protein | 24g |

## Includes

1 food from Column 1 & 1 food from Column 2

# Ray's Cheese Blintzes

A mouth-watering breakfast you can whip up with a couple of pan-cakes and some cottage cheese.

## Serves 1

## Ingredients

2   pancakes
    (follow directions for pancakes, but use 3 egg whites instead of 1 egg)
$1/2$  cup no-fat cottage cheese

## Preparation

☐   Place ½ cup no-fat cottage cheese between two 5-6" pancakes and microwave until cheese melts.

## Hint

Top with fruit and you have a complete meal!

## Per Serving

| | | | |
|---|---|---|---|
| Calories | 230 (8% from fat) | Fat | 2g |
| Carbohydrates | 28g | Protein | 25g |

## Includes

1 food from Column 1 & 1 food from Column 2

•

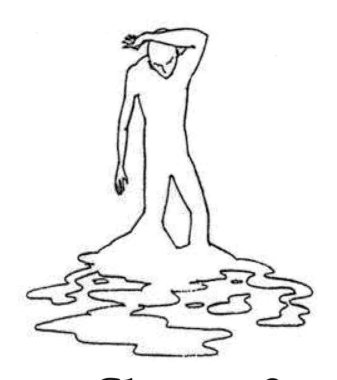

# Chapter 2
# Lunch
## Salads, Soups, Sandwiches and a few surprises!

# Dr. Jane's Salad Dressing

Creamy, peppery homemade dressing to spice up a quick salad. Nonfat yogurt provides calcium; horseradish and black pepper add flavor, without sodium. And best of all—you can prepare it in less than 10 minutes and store it in the refrigerator for up to 4 days!

## Makes 1½ cups

## Ingredients

| | |
|---|---|
| 1 | cup plain nonfat yogurt |
| 2 | tablespoons buttermilk |
| 2 | tablespoons nonfat mayonnaise |
| 1 | tablespoon grated white horseradish |
| 2 | teaspoons Dijon-style mustard |
| 1 | tablespoon chopped fresh parsley |
| 1 | teaspoon chopped fresh dill or ¼ teaspoon dried dillweed |
| ¼ | teaspoon celery seed |
| ¼ | teaspoon black pepper |

## Preparation

- In medium bowl, combine yogurt, buttermilk, and mayonnaise. Mix well. Add horseradish, parsley, dill, celery seed, and pepper. Mix well.
- Place the dressing in a serving bowl and serve immediately, or store in bowl covered with plastic wrap for up to 4 days.

## Try This

You can add or substitute other spices and herbs to the dressing.

## Hint

This dressing can be used on potatoes and veggies as well as salad with no guilt!

## Per Tablespoon

| | | | |
|---|---|---|---|
| Calories | 20 (36% from fat) | Fat | 1g |
| Carbohydrates | 2g | Protein | 1g |

# Waldorf Chicken Salad

Chicken turns this Waldorf Salad into a delicious and satisfying lunch that's quick to prepare!

## Serves 4

## Ingredients

| | |
|---|---|
| 4 | cups cooked, shredded chicken |
| 1 | cup chopped celery |
| 1 | medium Granny Smith or Red Delicious apple, unpeeled, thinly sliced (about 1 cup) |
| ½ | cup chopped walnuts |
| ½ | cup green onion |
| | Assorted lettuce leaves |

## Dresing

| | |
|---|---|
| 1 | cup fat-free mayonnaise |
| ½ | cup low-fat sour cream |
| 2 | tablespoons apple juice |
| ⅛ | teaspoon ground nutmeg |

## Preparation

- Prepare dressing in small bowl. Combine mayonnaise, sour cream, apple juice, and nutmeg and mix well.
- In large bowl combine chicken, celery, apple slices, walnuts, green onion and lettuce leaves. Pour dressing over salad and toss to coat.

## Try This

You can substitute turkey breast or reduced-sodium ham for the chicken. Chop turkey or ham into bite-size pieces.

## Hint

Just add a roll to make this lunch complete!

## Per Serving

| | | | | |
|---|---|---|---|---|
| Calories | 203 (26% from fat) | | Fat | 5g |
| Carbohydrates | 20g | | Protein | 20g |

## Includes

1 food from Column 2 & 1 food from Column 3 veggie list

# Chicken & Vegetable Salad

A great alternative to a leafy salad - a crunchy vegetable and chicken dish that's perfect for lunch or dinner. Vegetables are steamed to retain most of their nutrients. Carrots provide vitamin A.

## Serves 4

## Ingredients

| | |
|---|---|
| 3 | cups cooked cubed chicken |
| 1 | pound fresh green or yellow string beans, trimmed |
| 1 | small carrot (about ½ cup, julienned) |
| 1 | medium red or green bell pepper (about 1 cup), julienned |
| 1 | small red onion, thinly sliced (about ½ cup) |
| ¼ | cup nonfat Italian dressing |
| ½ | teaspoon freshly ground black pepper |

## Preparation

- Steam green beans and carrots until crisp-tender, about 4-5 minutes.
- In serving bowl combine chicken, bell pepper, onion, salad dressing, and black pepper. Mix well.
- Add green beans and carrots and toss gently to combine vegetables with dressing. Serve immediately.

## Try This

You can substitute turkey for the chicken - the perfect dish to make with leftovers.

## Hint

Just add a roll, and lunch will be complete!

## Per Serving

| | | | |
|---|---|---|---|
| Calories | 140 (12% from fat) | Fat | 2g |
| Carbohydrates | 15g | Protein | 18g |

## Includes

1 food from Column 2 & 1 food from Column 3 veggie list

# Turkey Salad Sandwich

Spicy turkey salad with sweet red peppers, corn and green onions. Colorful, crunchy and packed with vitamins.

## Makes 4 sandwiches

## Ingredients

| | |
|---|---|
| 2 | cups diced cooked turkey or chicken (8 ounces) |
| 1 | small sweet red pepper, finely chopped (½ cup) |
| ½ | cup frozen corn kernels, thawed and drained |
| 2 | green onions, including tops, sliced (¼ cup) |
| ½ | cup plain low-fat yogurt |
| ¾ | teaspoon ground cumin |
| ⅛ | teaspoon salt |
| 8 | slices whole-grain bread |

## Preparation

- In a large bowl, combine turkey, pepper, corn, green onions, yogurt, cumin and salt.
- Make four sandwiches using equal amounts of turkey salad. Cut each sandwich in half and serve.

## Hint

Munch on a few carrots to make this lunch a complete meal.

## Per Serving

| | | | | |
|---|---|---|---|---|
| Calories | 244 (11% from fat) | | Fat | 3g |
| Carbohydrates | 30g | | Protein | 24g |

## Includes

1 food from Column 1, 1 food from Column 2, ½ food from Column 3, & a Vegetable item.

# Mediterranean Style Chicken Soup

A colorful, chunky, hearty soup. Perfect to warm up a cold winter day!

## Serves 4

## Ingredients

| | |
|---|---|
| 1 | tablespoon olive oil |
| 2 | medium coarsely chopped yellow onions (about 1 cup) |
| 2 | medium coarsely chopped green bell peppers (about ¾ cup) |
| 2 | cloves minced garlic |
| 1 | can (14¼ ounces) low-sodium tomatoes, chopped, with their juice |
| 4 | cups low-sodium low-fat chicken broth |
| 2 | cups water |
| ¼ | cup long-grain white rice |
| 1 | tablespoon minced fresh basil (or 1 teaspoon dried basil, crumbled) |
| 6 | medium carrots, sliced ½ inch thick (about 4½ cups) |
| 1 | pound skinned and boned chicken breasts, cut into ¾-inch cubes |
| 1 | package (10 ounces) frozen green beans |
| ¼ | teaspoon black pepper |

## Preparation

- In a stockpot or 5-quart Dutch oven, heat olive oil over moderate heat. Add onion, green pepper and garlic; sauté, stirring occasionally for 5 minutes or until vegetables are soft.
- Stir in the tomatoes and their juice, the broth, water, rice and basil and bring to a boil. Lower heat to simmer mixture gently and cover and cook for 10 minutes. Add carrots and cook for 5 more minutes.
- Add chicken and green beans and cook uncovered for 5 minutes or until chicken is just cooked through. Stir in black pepper.

## Try This

This meal is complete as is. For a variation you can substitute skinless boneless turkey for the chicken. Try adding mushrooms or potatoes; they're low in sodium, high in potassium.

## Per Serving

| | | | |
|---|---|---|---|
| Calories | 336 (2% from fat) | Fat | 1g |
| Carbohydrates | 44g | Protein | 34g |

## Includes

1 serving from Column 1, 1 serving from Column 2 & 1 serving from Column 3

# Tasty Turkey Burgers

A great way to have that juicy burger without getting the fat. You can prepare and cook these tasty burgers in under 30 minutes!

## Serves 4

## Ingredients

| | |
|---|---|
| 1 | pound ground turkey (be sure turkey is low-fat) |
| 1 | small yellow onion, grated, drained and squeezed dry |
| 1 | tablespoon minced fresh sage or 1 teaspoon ground sage |
| ½ | cup soft whole-wheat bread crumbs |
| ¼ | teaspoon salt |
| ¼ | teaspoon pepper |

## Preparation

- Preheat broiler setting rack 6 inches from heat. In medium bowl combine turkey, sage, bread crumbs, salt and pepper. With moistened hands, form mixture into 4 patties.
- Place the patties on a lightly greased broiler pan and broil for 5 minutes. Turn patties over and broil 5 minutes more or until juices run clear when a patty is pricked with a fork.

## Hint

Include a roll and salad or veggies to make this meal complete.

## Per Serving

| | | | |
|---|---|---|---|
| Calories | 159 (22% from fat) | Fat | 4g |
| Carbohydrates | 5g | Protein | 26g |

## Includes

1 serving from Column 2

# Sweet Potato with Wings

This main-dish sweet potato salad with turkey is perfect for lunch or supper. A fantastic recipe to use up those holiday leftovers.

## Serves 4

## Ingredients

| | |
|---|---|
| 3 | tablespoons red currant jelly |
| ½ | cup low-sodium chicken broth |
| 1 | tablespoon lemon juice |
| 1 | tablespoon olive oil |
| ½ | teaspoon dried rosemary or savory, crumbled (or poultry seasoning) |
| ¼ | teaspoon salt |
| 12 | ounces cooked turkey, cut into ¾-inch cubes (about 3 cups) |
| 1 | large cooked sweet potato, peeled and cut into ¾-inch cubes (2 cups) |
| 1 | cup frozen corn kernels, rinsed under hot water and drained |
| 2 | green onions, thinly sliced (about ¼ cup) |
| 8 | romaine or red leaf lettuce leaves (optional) |

## Preparation

- In a large saucepan, warm the jelly and broth over moderate heat for about 2 minutes or until the jelly has melted. Whisk in the lemon juice, oil, rosemary, and salt.
- In a large bowl, combine the turkey, sweet potato, corn, and green onions. Add the dressing and toss until well coated. Place 2 lettuce leaves on each individual plate if desired, and spoon the salad on top.

## Hint

Add some raw carrots, broccoli, and peppers to complete this meal.

## Per Serving

| | | | |
|---|---|---|---|
| Calories | 410 (15% from fat) | Fat | 7g |
| Carbohydrates | 59g | Protein | 30g |

## Includes

1 food from Column 1 & 1 food from Column 2

# Chicken Tortillas

Enjoy these tortillas hot or at room temperature. Great with tomato salsa!

## Serves 6

## Ingredients

| | |
|---|---|
| 6 | flour tortillas, 7 inches in diameter |
| 2 | cups diced cooked chicken or turkey (8 ounces) |
| ½ | cup shredded low-fat Monterey Jack cheese |
| 1 | small red onion, finely chopped (about ½ cup) |
| ½ | cup drained, chopped roasted sweet red peppers |
| 1 | can (4 ounces) chopped green chilies, drained |
| 1 | clove garlic, minced |
| 1 | teaspoon ground cumin |
| 2 | tablespoons minced parsley mixed with ¾ teaspoon dried cilantro |

## Preparation

- Preheat oven to 400° F. Wrap the tortillas in aluminum foil and heat in the oven for 5 minutes or until warm. Preheat broiler, setting rack 6 inches from heat.
- Combine chicken, cheese, onions, peppers, chilies, garlic, cumin and cilantro in medium size bowl. Spread equal amount of mixture in the center of each tortilla, then fold the tortilla in half to enclose filling
- Transfer tortillas to baking sheet. Broil for 2½ to 3 minutes on each side until crisp and blistered. Serve immediately.

## Try This

You can refrigerate the broiled tortillas and use them another day. Wrap them in aluminum foil and refrigerate for up to 2 days, letting them come to room temperature before serving.

## Hint

This meal is almost complete. Just add a salad to make it complete!

## Per Serving

| | | | | |
|---|---|---|---|---|
| Calories | 280 (16% from fat) | | Fat | 5g |
| Carbohydrates | 21g | | Protein | 19g |

## Includes

1 food from Column 1, 1 food from Column 2 & ½ food from Column 3

# Tuna Niçoise Pitas

Red Leaf lettuce is low-cal, high in fiber and a good source of Vitamin A. Tuna is a great source of protein.

## Serves 2

## Ingredients

| | |
|---|---|
| 1 | cup frozen cut green beans |
| 1 | can (6½ ounces) tuna packed in water, drained |
| 2 | plum tomatoes, diced |
| 4 | black olives (preferably Niçoise or Calamata), pitted, finely chopped |
| 2 | tablespoons finely chopped red onion |
| 2 | tablespoons snipped fresh dill or minced fresh basil or parsley |
| 1 | teaspoon olive oil |
| 2 | tablespoons lemon juice |
| ⅛ | teaspoon black pepper, or to taste |
| 2 | whole-wheat pita rounds, halved |

Lettuce Leaves (preferably red leaf or Boston)

## Preparation

- Steam green beans until tender.
- In large bowl, mix tuna, green beans, tomatoes, olives, onions, dill, oil, lemon juice, and pepper. Place several lettuce leaves into each pita half, then fill with the Tuna Niçoise.

## Try This

You can also use chicken or turkey in the filling. Or for a great seafood pocket substitute salmon.

## Hint

This lunch is complete - don't worry about the extra protein.

## Per Serving

| | | | |
|---|---|---|---|
| Calories | 300 (15% from fat) | Fat | 5g |
| Carbohydrates | 34g | Protein | 32g |

## Includes

1 food from Column 1, 1½ foods from Column 2 & 1 food from Column 3

# Elaine's Fried Rice

Cook up some lean meat ahead of time, or use up those leftovers in the fridge to make this quick delicious meal.

## Serves 4

## Ingredients

| | |
|---|---|
| ½ | cup chopped onion |
| 4 | tablespoons chopped green pepper |
| 1 | tablespoon canola oil |
| 4 | cups cooked rice |
| 1 | teaspoon olive oil |
| 2 | five ounce cans sliced,drained water chestnuts |
| 6 | ounces sliced mushrooms |
| 4 | tablespoons soy sauce |
| 1 | cup cooked chicken, shrimp or lean meat |
| 1½ | cup egg substitute |

## Preparation

- In large skillet, cook and stir onion and green pepper in oil until onion is tender.
- Stir in rice, water chestnuts, mushrooms, and soy sauce. Cook over low heat 10 minutes, stirring frequently.
- Add meat, chicken, or shrimp and heat through. Stir in egg substitute; cook and stir 2 to 3 minutes longer.

## Hint

To complete this lunch, just add veggies or a salad.

## Per Serving

| | | | |
|---|---|---|---|
| Calories | 275 (15% from fat) | Fat | 4.5g |
| Carbohydrates | 38g | Protein | 21g |

## Includes

1 food from Column 1 & 1food from Column 2

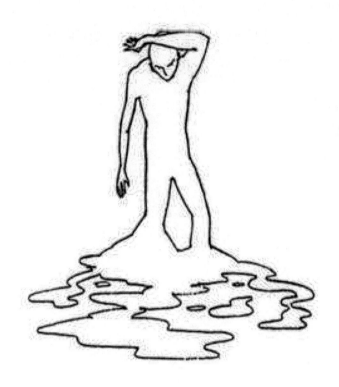

# Chapter 3
# Dinner
# Fish

# Fish Fillets

These fillets are crisp on the outside, moist on the inside. "Oven-fried" fish to give you that deep fried taste without the fat. Prepare and cook it in under 30 minutes!

## Serves 4

## Ingredients

| | |
|---|---|
| ¼ | cup fresh bread crumbs |
| ¼ | cup yellow cornmeal |
| ½ | teaspoon paprika |
| ½ | teaspoon dried thyme |
| ¼ | teaspoon grated lemon peel |
| ¼ | teaspoon salt |
| ⅛ | teaspoon black pepper |
| 1 | egg white |
| 4 | cod, scrod, or haddock fillets (about 5 ounces each) |

Lemon wedges and fresh thyme sprigs for garnish

## Preparation

☐ Preheat oven to 425° F. Place oven rack on lowest level. Spray a nonstick baking sheet with vegetable cooking spray. Set aside.

☐ On a sheet of waxed paper, combine the bread crumbs, cornmeal, paprika, dried thyme, lemon peel, salt, and pepper. Mix well.

☐ In a shallow bowl, lightly beat egg white, draining off excess, then dredge in bread crumb mixture, turning to coat. Place on prepared baking sheet.

☐ Bake until bottom of fish is golden brown, about 7 minutes. Turn fillets and bake until just cooked, about 5 to 6 minutes. Garnish with lemon wedges and thyme, serve.

## Try This:

This recipe works great with shrimp too! Substitute 1¼ pounds of shelled medium shrimp for fillets and use ½ teaspoon of dried tarragon instead of thyme. Reduce cooking time to 5 minutes each side.

## Hint

To complete this meal, add baked french fries (see Guiltless Fish & Chips) and cole slaw made with low-fat dressing.

## Per Serving

| | | | |
|---|---|---|---|
| Calories | 163 (8% from fat) | Fat | 1g |
| Carbohydrates | 8g | Protein | 27g |

## Includes

1 food from Column 2

# Fiesta Pasta & Tuna Salad

Tricolor corkscrew pasta and tuna provide a colorful, festive, cool salad dish with carbs, protein and low fat. Prepare and cook in 30 minutes!

## Serves 4

## Ingredients

| | |
|---|---|
| 8 | ounces tricolor corkscrew pasta |
| 16 | ounces green beans, trimmed and cut into 2-inch pieces |
| 1 | medium red onion, thinly sliced (about 1 cup) |
| $^2/_3$ | cup reduced-fat Italian salad dressing |
| ¼ | cup chopped fresh parsley |
| ¼ | cup chopped fresh basil |
| 1 | cup cherry tomatoes cut in half |
| 2 | cans (6⅛ ounces each) tuna packed in water, drained and flaked |

Fresh basil sprigs for garnish

## Preparation

- Cook pasta according to package directions, but eliminate salt. About 7 minutes before pasta is done, add green beans to pot. Remove pot from heat and add onion. Drain in colander and rinse under cold water. Drain again.
- While pasta mixture is draining, combine dressing, parsley, and chopped basil in large serving bowl. Mix well
- Add pasta mixture to dressing mixture. Add tomatoes and tuna. Toss to coat. Garnish with basil sprigs and serve.

## Hint

This recipe provides a complete meal.

## Per Serving

| | | | |
|---|---|---|---|
| Calories | 361 (10% from fat) | Fat | 4g |
| Carbohydrates | 54g | Protein | 27g |

## Includes

1 food from Column 1, 1 food from Column 2 & 1 food from Column 3 veggie list

# Tangy Tex Mex Fish Cakes

Cod never tasted so good - jalapeño peppers and cilantro add a zing, but few calories. Served with salsa, a low-sodium treat.

## Serves 4

## Ingredients

| | |
|---|---|
| ½ | cup all-purpose flour |
| 2 | cups mashed potatoes, cooled |
| 1 | pound cooked cod fish, cooled and flaked |
| 2 | tablespoons chopped fresh cilantro |
| 1 | teaspoon minced jalapeño pepper |
| ½ | teaspoon dried onion flakes |
| ½ | teaspoon salt |
| ½ | teaspoon freshly ground black pepper |
| 1 | egg white, lightly beaten |
| ½ | cup cornmeal |
| 1 | cup prepared salsa |

## Preparation

- Spray a baking sheet with vegetable cooking spray. Spread flour on a sheet of waxed paper.
- In a large bowl, combine potatoes, fish, cilantro, jalapeño pepper, onion flakes, salt, and black pepper. Mix well.
- Divide fish mixture into 9 equal mounds. Shape each into a round cake. Dredge in flour. Dip into egg white, allowing excess to drip into bowl. Dredge in cornmeal, patting to cover well.
- Place fish cakes on prepared baking sheet; chill for 10 minutes before baking to help fish cakes hold their shape. Preheat oven to 375° F.
- Bake, turning once, until golden, about 30 minutes. Place fish cakes on plates and serve with salsa. Serve immediately.

## Hint

To complete this meal, simply add a salad or roasted peppers.

## Per Serving

| | | | |
|---|---|---|---|
| Calories | 325 (7% from fat) | Fat | 2g |
| Carbohydrates | 45g | Protein | 32g |

## Includes

1 food from Column 1 & 1½ foods from Column 2

# Guiltless Fish and Chips

Low-fat batter-dipped fish with a side of fries. Use cod or haddock as a very low-fat fish choice. Skins on potatoes provide extra fiber.

## Serves 4

## Ingredients

| | |
|---|---|
| $\frac{1}{8}$ | cup bread crumbs |
| $\frac{1}{2}$ | teaspoon freshly ground black pepper |
| $\frac{1}{4}$ | teaspoon salt |
| 1 | egg white, lightly beaten |
| 1 | pound cod or haddock fillets, cut into 1½-inch-wide strips |
| 1 | tablespoon olive oil |

## For the Chips

| | |
|---|---|
| 2 | medium russet potatoes |
| 1 | tablespoon olive oil |
| $\frac{1}{4}$ | teaspoon salt |

## Preparation

- Preheat oven to 450° F. Spray a large shallow baking pan with vegetable cooking spray.
- To prepare chips, cut potatoes lengthwise into 1-inch strips. Place in large bowl, toss with oil and salt. Arrange chips on prepared pan and bake until golden brown, turning once, about 30 minutes.
- While chips are baking, on a sheet of wax paper, combine bread crumbs, pepper and salt. Mix well.
- Place egg white in a shallow dish. Dip fish into egg white, allowing excess to drip back into dish. Dredge fish in bread crumb mixture; pat to coat fish thoroughly on all sides.
- In a large skillet, heat oil over medium-high heat. Add some fish to skillet. Cook until golden and fish flakes easily when tested with a fork, about 5 minutes. Drain on paper towels; cover with foil to keep warm. Repeat with remaining fish. Serve immediately with chips.

## Hint

A roll and cole slaw with low-fat dressing will complete this meal.

## Per Serving

| | | | |
|---|---|---|---|
| Calories | 253 (29% from fat) | Fat | 8g |
| Carbohydrates | 20g | Protein | 25g |

## Includes

½ food from Column 1 and 1 food from Column 2

# Shrimp Gumbo

A southern dish served up with shrimp, chicken, and very little fat! Shrimp is a low-fat, low-sodium treat. Filé powder, a Cajun seasoning, can be added to enhance the taste and body of gumbos.

## Serves 4

## Ingredients

| | |
|---|---|
| 1 | tablespoon olive oil |
| ½ | cup (about 1 small) onion, chopped |
| ¼ | cup chopped green bell pepper |
| ½ | cup peeled, seeded, chopped plum tomatoes |
| 3 | cloves garlic, minced |
| 4 | cups reduced-sodium chicken broth |
| ½ | teaspoon hot pepper sauce |
| 2 | cups sliced fresh or frozen okra |
| 1 | pound medium shrimp, peeled and deveined (or any white fish) |
| 1 | teaspoon filé powder (optional) |

## Preparation

- In a large saucepan, heat oil over medium heat until hot but not smoking. Add onion and pepper to pan; sauté until vegetables are tender, about 7 minutes. Add tomatoes and garlic. Cook for 4 minutes, stir occasionally. Add broth and hot pepper sauce; cook for 10 minutes.
- Add okra; reduce heat to low. Add shrimp and simmer until shrimp turns pink, about 5 minutes. Stir in filé powder. Stir constantly and cook until mixture thickens, about 2 minutes.

## Hint

A roll of crackers will complete this meal.

## Per Serving

| | | | |
|---|---|---|---|
| Calories | 170 (18% from fat) | Fat | 3g |
| Carbohydrates | 15g | Protein | 21g |

## Includes

1 food from Column 2 and 1 food from Column 3 veggies list

# Garlic Scallop Kebabs

Maximum flavor achieved with very little fat or sodium. Scallops are a fantastic low-fat choice. Lemon juice, chicken broth, and garlic make these kebabs a flavor-packed meal. Peppers, onions and mushrooms (for protein and B vitamins) make a healthy, colorful and delicious accompaniment.

## Serves 6

## Ingredients

| | |
|---|---|
| $\frac{1}{3}$ | cup fresh lemon juice |
| $\frac{1}{3}$ | cup dry white wine or reduced-sodium chicken broth |
| 4 | cloves garlic, minced |
| 2 | bay leaves |
| 1 | teaspoon grated lemon peel |
| 1 | teaspoon black pepper |
| 1½ | pounds sea scallops |
| 4 | cups large mushroom caps |
| 3 | medium red bell peppers, cut into 1-inch squares (about 3 cups) |
| 3 | medium green bell peppers, cut into 1-inch squares (about 3 cups) |
| 2 | large red onions, cut into 1-inch squares (about 3 cups) |

## Preparation

- In a shallow glass dish, combine lemon juice, wine, garlic, bay leaves, lemon peel, and pepper and mix well. Reserve 3 tablespoons. Add scallops to dish; toss to coat. Cover dish with plastic wrap and refrigerate for 1 hour.
- Heat charcoal grill, preheat gas grill to medium, or preheat boiler. Spray grill rack or broiler pan with vegetable cooking spray.
- Remove scallops from marinade. Discard marinade in dish. Use six 12-inch metal skewers. Alternately thread scallops, mushrooms, bell peppers and onions. Place kebabs on prepared rack or pan.
- Grill or broil 6 inches from heat, turning occasionally and basting with reserved lemon mixture, until scallops are cooked through and vegetables are lightly browned, about 7 to 8 minutes. Serve immediately.

## Hint

A roll or crackers will complete this meal.

## Per Serving

| | | | |
|---|---|---|---|
| Calories | 190 (8% from fat) | Fat | 2g |
| Carbohydrates | 21g | Protein | 23g |

## Includes

1 food from Column 2 and 1 food from Column 3 veggie list

# Elaine's Easy Shrimp Dish

A shrimp dish that's quick to prepare!

## Serves 4

## Ingredients

| | |
|---|---|
| 16 | ounces large cooked shrimp |
| 1 | tablespoon lemon juice |
| 1 | tablespoon dry sherry |
| 1 | clove garlic, minced |
| 4 | tablespoons plain dried bread crumbs |
| 1 | ounce shredded cheese |
| 1 | tablespoon chopped fresh parsley |
| $\frac{1}{8}$ | teaspoon salt |
| dash | of pepper |

## Preparation

- Arrange shrimp in baking dish. Sprinkle lemon juice, sherry, and garlic over shrimp.
- Spread bread crumbs and cheese over shrimp. Top with parsley, salt, and pepper.
- Heat in 350° F. oven until warmed (about 15 minutes), then broil for 2 to 3 minutes until slightly browned.

## Hint

To complete this meal, serve with rice and add your favorite veggie from Column 3.

## Includes

1 food from Column 2

## Per Serving

| | | | |
|---|---|---|---|
| Calories | 122 (22% from fat) | Fat | 3g |
| Carbohydrates | 3g | Protein | 21g |

## Includes

1 food from Column 2

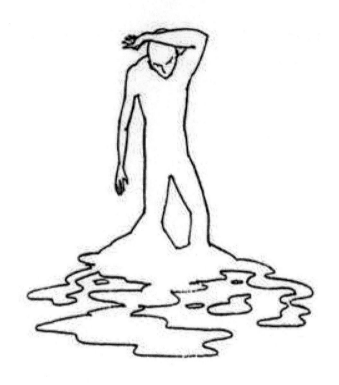

# Chapter 4
# Dinner
# Chicken & Turkey

# Chicken, Greens, and Sweet Potato Stew

## Serves 4

## Ingredients

| | |
|---|---|
| ¼ | cup all-purpose flour |
| 2 | tablespoons cornmeal |
| 1 | broiler-fryer (2 pounds), skinned and cut into 4 serving pieces |
| 2 | cups low-sodium chicken broth |
| 3 | medium sweet potatoes (1 pound), peeled and cut into 1-inch cubes |
| 6 | cloves garlic, slivered |
| 2 | tablespoons slivered fresh ginger |
| 1 | pound kale, spinach, or mustard or collard greens, rinsed, stems removed, and torn into bite-size pieces |

## Preparation

☐ On a sheet of wax paper, combine the flour and cornmeal. Dredge the chicken in the mixture, shaking off any excess. Spray a 5-quart Dutch oven with vegetable oil cooking spray. Over moderately high heat sauté chicken for about 3 minutes on each side or until golden brown.

☐ Add the stock, potatoes, garlic, and ginger and bring to a boil. Lower the heat and simmer, covered, for 20 minutes. Place the kale on top of the chicken and potatoes, cover and cook 5 minutes longer or until kale is tender and the chicken is cooked through.

## Hint

This meal is complete as is.

## Per Serving

| | | | | |
|---|---|---|---|---|
| Calories | 419 (11% from fat) | | Fat | 5g |
| Carbohydrates | 32g | | Protein | 44g |

## Includes

1 food from Column 1, 2 foods from Column 2 & ½ food from Column 3

# Chicken Tetrazzini

Serve up a mouth-watering dish of chicken, linguine, mushroom and peas covered with a light, creamy sauce made with skim milk and reduced sodium broth.

## Serves 4

## Ingredients

| | |
|---|---|
| 1 | tablespoon olive oil |
| 4 | skinless, boneless chicken breasts (3 ounces each) cut into 2" pieces |
| 8 | ounces linguine pasta |
| 1 | tablespoon margarine |
| 2 | tablespoons all-purpose flour |
| 1½ | cups skim milk |
| ⅓ | cup reduced sodium chicken broth |
| 2 | cups sliced mushrooms |
| ½ | cup thawed frozen peas |
| 2 | tablespoons chopped fresh parsley |
| ⅛ | teaspoon black pepper |

## Preparation

- Heat oil in large nonstick skillet over medium-high heat. Add chicken and cook (turning once) about 10 minutes, until no longer pink. While chicken is cooking, cook pasta according to package directions (do not add salt).
- Remove chicken from skillet; place on plate and cover with foil to keep warm.
- In same skillet, melt margarine over medium heat. Add flour and stir constantly for 2 minutes. Whisk milk and chicken broth into skillet. Add mushrooms and cook approximately 5 minutes, stirring frequently. Sauce should be slightly thick and the mushrooms, tender.
- Return chicken to skillet. Stir in peas, parsley, and pepper. Heat, stirring frequently, for 1 minute.
- Drain pasta in a colander. Place pasta on serving plates and spoon mixture over pasta. Serve immediately.

## Hint

To complete this meal, serve with a salad or cooked veggies.

## Per Serving

| | | | |
|---|---|---|---|
| Calories | 379 (19% from fat) | Fat | 8g |
| Carbohydrates | 36g | Protein | 38g |

## Includes

1 food from Column 1, 1½ foods from Column 2 and ½ food from Column 3 veggies

# Savory Chicken Stew

Simmer up a hearty hot stew in just three quarters of an hour, not a day! Skinless chicken breasts keep the fat count low; carrots are an excellent source of vitamin A.

## Serves 6

## Ingredients

| | |
|---|---|
| 1 | 28-ounce can Italian-style tomatoes, undrained |
| 1 | can (13¾ ounces) reduced-sodium chicken broth |
| 6 | skinless, boneless chicken breast halves (4 oz ea), cut into ¾" cubes |
| 3 | medium russet potatoes, peeled and cut into ½" cubes (about 3 cups) |
| 2 | large yellow onions, chopped (about 2½ cups) |
| 1 | cup chopped celery |
| 1 | tablespoon chopped fresh marjoram or 1 teaspoon dried marjoram |
| ½ | teaspoon freshly ground black pepper |
| 2 | packages (20 ounces) carrots |

## Preparation

- In a 5-quart Dutch oven, combine tomatoes and broth and bring to a boil over high heat.
- Add the chicken, potatoes, onions, celery, chopped marjoram, and pepper and return to a boil. Reduce heat to low; cover and simmer for 10 minutes
- Add carrots and return to a boil. Cover and reduce heat to low. Simmer until vegetables are fork-tender, about 10 minutes.
- Serve immediately, garnished with parsley or marjoram sprigs.

## Try This

You can place the cooked stew into a bowl, cover with plastic wrap and refrigerate for up to a day. To reheat, place in a Dutch oven over medium-low heat and simmer until heated through.

## Hint

This meal is complete as is.

## Per Serving

| | | | |
|---|---|---|---|
| Calories | 300 (7% from fat) | Fat | 2g |
| Carbohydrates | 35g | Protein | 33g |

## Includes

1 food from Column 1, 1 food from Column 2 and 1food from Column 3, veggies

# Chicken Stir-Fry

Tender chicken served with crisp vegetables provides a meal that's high in protein and vitamins A and D and low in fat and sodium.

## Serves 4

## Ingredients

| | |
|---|---|
| ¼ | cup orange juice |
| 1½ | tablespoons cornstarch |
| 1 | pound skinless, boneless chicken breasts, cut into strips |
| ¾ | cup reduced-sodium chicken broth |
| 1½ | tablespoons reduced-sodium soy sauce |
| 2½ | teaspoons olive oil |
| 1 | clove garlic, minced |
| 1 | tablespoon minced fresh ginger or 1½ teaspoons ground ginger |
| 2 | cups green beans |
| 1 | medium red bell pepper, cut into thin strips (about 1 cup) |
| ¾ | cup sliced green onion |
| 2 | cups cooked white rice |

## Preparation

- Combine orange juice and cornstarch in shallow glass bowl and mix well. Stir in chicken. Cover bowl with plastic wrap and refrigerate for 2 hours.
- Drain chicken and discard mixture. In small bowl, combine broth and soy sauce; set aside
- Heat oil over medium heat in a wok or large skillet. Add garlic and ginger; stir-fry for 30 seconds. Add chicken; stir-fry for 3 minutes. Add vegetables; stir fry about 5 minutes until crisp-tender. Stir in broth mixture.
- Place ½ cup of rice on each plate. Top with the chicken mixture.

## Hint

Here's another complete meal as is.

## Per Serving

| | | | |
|---|---|---|---|
| Calories | 368 (13% from fat) | Fat | 5g |
| Carbohydrates | 43g | Protein | 31g |

## Includes

1 serving from Column 1, 1 serving from Column 2 and 1 serving from Column 3

# Chicken and Couscous

For a change of pace, try couscous, small grains of semolina pasta, instead of rice; it's a good source of complex carbohydrates and makes a delicious side dish to chicken.

## Serves 6

## Ingredients

| | |
|---|---|
| 1½ | teaspoons ground cumin |
| ¼ | teaspoon ground cinnamon |
| ¼ | teaspoon salt |
| ⅛ | teaspoon cayenne pepper |
| 6 | skinless, boneless chicken thighs (5 ounces each) |
| 2 | medium sweet potatoes, peeled and cut into 1" cubes (about 2 cups) |
| 3 | cloves garlic, minced |
| 2½ | cups water |
| 1 | cup couscous |
| 2 | tablespoons fresh lemon juice |

Chopped fresh mint for garnish

## Preparation

- Preheat oven to 375° F. Combine cumin, cinnamon, salt, and cayenne pepper in a small bowl and mix well.
- Trim visible fat from chicken thighs. Rub some of spice mixture onto each thigh, fold flaps of thighs under, and set chicken aside. Reserve remaining spice mixture.
- In medium ovenproof casserole dish, combine sweet potatoes, garlic, and remaining spice mixture. Mix well, top with chicken, and add enough water to cover.
- Bring casserole to a boil over high heat; cover and place in oven. Bake about 25 minutes until chicken is cooked through and sweet potatoes are tender.
- Remove casserole from oven; sprinkle couscous on top, pushing it into liquid with a spoon. Cover and let stand until liquid is absorbed, about 5 to 10 minutes. Drizzle with lemon juice, garnish with mint and serve immediately. Hint: Serve with green beans to make a complete meal.

## Per Serving

| | | | |
|---|---|---|---|
| Calories | 356 (15% from fat) | Fat | 6g |
| Carbohydrates | 41g | Protein | 33g |

## Includes

1 serving from Column 1 and 1½ serving from Column 2

# Chicken Fajitas

Tex-Mex tortillas stuffed with chicken and fresh vegetables provide you with iron and protein. Flour tortillas are low in fat. Chicken is broiled to seal in flavor and reduce fat; red bell peppers and lime juice add a sweet and zesty fat-free taste.

## Serves 4

## Ingredients

| | |
|---|---|
| ¼ | teaspoons olive oil |
| 2 | teaspoons olive oil |
| ½ | teaspoon chili powder |
| ½ | teaspoon ground cumin |
| 4 | skinless, boneless chicken breast halves (4 ounces each) |
| 2 | medium red bell peppers, cut into wide strips (about 2 cups) |
| 1 | large red onion, cut into wedges (about 1½ cups) |
| 2 | medium tomatoes, chopped (about 2 cups), divided |
| ½ | cup chopped green onion |
| ¼ | cup chopped fresh cilantro or parsley, divided |
| 8 | flour tortillas, warmed |

## Preparation

- ☐ Combine lime juice, oil, and spices in shallow glass dish and mix well. Reserve 2 tablespoons of marinade. Add chicken to dish; turn to coat. Cover dish with plastic wrap and refrigerate 30 minutes.
- ☐ Preheat broiler. Drain the chicken and discard marinade. Place on broiler pan and broil three inches from heat, basting with the reserved marinade. Cook about 10 minutes, turning once, until no longer pink in center. Place chicken on a plate; cover to keep warm.
- ☐ Place bell peppers and red onion on broiler pan. Broil until lightly charred, turning once, about 8 minutes.
- ☐ Cut chicken into strips; place in a large bowl. Add broiled vegetables, 1 cup of tomatoes, green onion, and 2 tablespoons of cilantro. Mix gently. Top tortillas with chicken mixture and fold to enclose filling. Serve with remaining tomatoes and cilantro.

## Hint

Here's a great meal that's complete as is.

## Per Serving

| | | | |
|---|---|---|---|
| Calories | 426 (19% from fat) | Fat | 8g |
| Carbohydrates | 60g | Protein | 30g |

## Includes

1 serving from Column 1, 1 serving from Column 2 and 1 serving from Column 3 veggie list

# Roast Chicken

A flavorful main dish served with vegetables and prepared with herbs to enhance flavor and provide fiber without adding fat. Turnips are low in calories and high in vitamin C.

## Serves 4

## Ingredients

| | |
|---|---|
| 2 | teaspoons olive oil |
| 1 | clove garlic, peeled |
| 4 | skinless, boneless chicken breast halves (4 ounces each) |
| ¼ | teaspoon paprika |
| ⅛ | teaspoon black pepper |
| 3 | cups 1-inch carrot pieces |
| 2 | cups 1-inch turnip pieces |
| ½ | cup reduced-sodium chicken broth |
| 2 | tablespoons chopped fresh oregano or 2 teaspoons dried oregano |

Fresh oregano sprigs for garnish

## Preparation

- Preheat oven to 400° F. Heat oil in large ovenproof nonstick skillet over medium-low heat. Add garlic and sauté for 3 minutes. Remove garlic and discard.
- Increase heat to medium-high. Sprinkle chicken with paprika and pepper. Add to skillet; sauté until golden, turning once, about 2 minutes per side. Transfer the chicken to a plate; set aside.
- Add carrots, turnip, broth, and chopped oregano to skillet. Cook for 5 minutes. Return chicken and any juices from plate to pan. Cover skillet with foil.
- Place skillet in oven; bake until chicken is no longer pink in center and vegetables are tender, about 20 to 25 minutes. Garnish with oregano sprigs and serve. Hint: Simply serve with potatoes or rolls to complete this meal.

## Try This

Chicken breasts may be sliced into 1-inch strips and vegetables diced to reduce cooking time. Follow recipe but decrease baking time to about 15 minutes.

## Per Serving

| | | | |
|---|---|---|---|
| Calories | 239 (8% from fat) | Fat | 2g |
| Carbohydrates | 25g | Protein | 29g |

## Includes

1 serving from Column 2 and 1 serving from Column 3, veggies

# Dr. Dalpe's Turkey Chili

Hot and spicy chili made with turkey to reduce fat content. Peppers and kidney beans are an excellent source of fiber.

## Serves 4

## Ingredients

| | |
|---|---|
| 2 | teaspoons olive oil |
| 1 | medium yellow onion, finely chopped (about 1 cup) |
| 1 | large sweet green pepper, diced (about 1 cup) |
| 1 | pound ground low fat turkey |
| 2 | teaspoons each ground cumin and chili powder |
| ¼ | teaspoon salt |
| 2 | cloves garlic, minced |
| 1 | can (14½ ounces) low-sodium tomatoes, chopped, with their juice |
| ½ | teaspoon each dried basil and oregano, crumbled |
| 1½ | cups cooked red kidney beans |
| 1 | tablespoon minced fresh cilantro (coriander) (optional garrnish) |

## Preparation

- Heat oil in 12-inch nonstick skillet over moderate heat. Add onion and green pepper and sauté, stirring occasionally, for 5 minutes or until onion is softened. Add turkey and sauté 3 minutes or until turkey is no longer pink. Add cumin, chili powder, salt, and garlic and sauté, stirring, 1 minute more.
- Stir in the tomatoes, basil, and oregano and lower the heat. Simmer and stir occasionally for 20 minutes. Stir in the beans and simmer 5 to 7 minutes more until beans are heated through. If desired, garnish with cilantro. Serve with rice and a lettuce and tomato salad.

## Hint

If you like chili, you'll love this version. Simply add another large pepper to complete this meal.

## Per Serving

| | | | | |
|---|---|---|---|---|
| Calories | 283 (12% from fat) | | Fat | 6g |
| Carbohydrates | 25g | | Protein | 38g |

## Includes

1 food from Column 1, 2 foods from Column 2 and ½ food from Column 3

# Chicken Black Bean Soup

## Serves 4

## Ingredients

¼     cup dried black beans
2     cups water
1     bay leaf
Light vegetable oil cooking spray
½     cup peeled and chopped broccoli stems
½     cup scraped and cubed carrot (1 medium carrot)
1     cup scraped and cubed celery (2 medium stalks)
1     cup chopped onion (1 medium onion)
1     tablespoon dried thyme
1     tablespoon dried basil
½     cup dry white wine
8     ounces boneless, skinless chicken breast
4     tablespoons barbecue sauce (no-oil variety)
1     cup chicken stock, fat skimmed off
12     ounces evaporated skim milk
2     cups broccoli florets (1 bundle)
1     tablespoon cornstarch dissolved in 2 tablespoons cold water
1     tablespoon Worcestershire sauce
1     teaspoon Tabasco sauce
¼     cup chopped fresh cilantro

## Preparation

- Pick over and rinse the beans. Put them into a large bowl and cover completely with cold water. Let the beans soak overnight (or at least 8 hours).
- Drain the beans and transfer them to a medium saucepan. Add the 2 cups water and the bay leaf. Bring to a boil over medium heat and cool for 15 minutes. Reduce the heat to low and simmer, uncovered, for about 20 minutes, until the beans are tender. Drain the beans and discard the bay leaf.

(Continued on next page.)

# Chicken Black Bean Soup (Cont'd)

- ☐ Preheat oven to 400 degrees.
- ☐ Place a heavy stockpot over medium heat for about 1 minute, then spray it twice with the vegetable oil. Add broccoli stems, carrot, celery, and onion. Cover and reduce heat to low; cook for 5 minutes, stirring once or twice. Stir in the thyme, basil, and wine. Simmer, uncovered, for about 15 minutes, until the wine has been reduced by half.
- ☐ In the meantime, coat the chicken thoroughly with the barbecue sauce and bake for 10 minutes on the top shelf of the oven. Remove the chicken from the oven and allow it to cool just long enough to handle. Cut the chicken into small cubes.
- ☐ Add the chicken, chicken stock, and beans to the stockpot. Cook over low heat for about 3 minutes until thoroughly heated. Stir in the evaporated milk and the broccoli florets. Cook for 5 minutes, stirring if needed to keep the soup from coming to a boil. Add the dissolved cornstarch and cook for 2 minutes more, stirring constantly. Stir in the Worcestershire sauce, and Tabasco sauce.
- ☐ Garnish with the chopped cilantro.

## Hint

This great meal is complete as is.

## Per Serving

| | | | |
|---|---|---|---|
| Calories | 368 (9% from fat) | Fat | 3.6g |
| Carbohydrates | 60g | Protein | 23g |

## Includes

1 food from Column 1, 1 food from Column 2 and 1 food from Column 3

# Tropical Chicken Salad

Serve this fruity chicken salad with Raspberry Vinaigrette Dressing. Don't mix the salad ingredients until just before serving—the enzyme in papaya breaks down the fiber in chicken and makes it very soft.

## Serves 6

## Ingredients

| | |
|---|---|
| $1/3$ | cup thinly sliced red onion |
| 7 | cups torn assorted salad green, rinsed and dried |
| 2 | cups diced cooked chicken breast meat (about 12 oz, from 2 breasts) |
| 1½ | cups bite-size mango pieces |
| 1½ | cups bite-size papaya pieces |

Cains Fat Free Raspberry Vinaigrette Dressing

## Preparation

☐ Place the onion slices in a bowl with cold water to cover and let them stand for 30 minutes. Drain the slices and pat them dry with paper toweling.

☐ Place the greens, chicken, mango, papaya, and onion in a large salad bowl. Pour the dressing over and toss to coat all the ingredients. Serve the salad immediately.

## Hint

This meal is easy to complete—just add a roll!

## Per Serving

| | | | |
|---|---|---|---|
| Calories | 130 (14% from fat) | Fat | 2g |
| Carbohydrates | 16g | Protein | 18g |

## Includes

½ food from Column 1, 1 food from Column 2 and 2 foods from Column 3

# Sue's Grilled Chicken & Broccoli in Red Sauce

Grilled chicken in tomato sauce with fresh vegetables gives this healthy dish a unique flavor.

## Serves 4

## Ingredients

| | |
|---|---|
| 1 | teaspoon olive oil |
| 1 | pound boneless, skinless chicken grilled and sliced into strips |
| 1 | 28 ounce can No Salt Added Whole tomatoes undrained & chopped |
| 4-6 | plum tomatoes coarsely chopped |
| 2 | cups broccoli florets |
| 1 | cup fresh sliced mushrooms |
| 3 | tablespoons fresh chopped parsley |
| 4-5 | cloves fresh garlic thinly sliced |
| 8 | black olives sliced in half |

Fresh basil, chopped
Salt and pepper to taste

## Preparation

- Combine canned and fresh tomatoes, parsley, salt, and fresh ground pepper in a bowl; set aside. (This can be done several hours ahead.)
- Sauté garlic in olive oil until fragrant. Add tomato mixture, bring to a boil.
- Add chicken pieces, broccoli, mushrooms, and olives and simmer approximately 15 minutes until vegetables are cooked but still firm.
- Serve over pasta, sprinkle with fresh basil.

## Try This

Grilled shrimp can be substituted for chicken for a great-tasting seafood dinner.

## Hint

Here's another great meal that's complete when served over pasta.

## Per Serving

| | | | |
|---|---|---|---|
| Calories | 250 (23% from fat) | Fat | 6.5g |
| Carbohydrates | 11g | Protein | 37g |

## Includes

1 food from Column 2 and 1 food from Column 3

# Chicken Fajita Salad

If you like fajitas, you'll love this low cal salad. Chicken is broiled to seal in flavor and reduce fat; red bell peppers and lime juice add a sweet and zesty fat-free taste.

## Serves 4

## Ingredients

| | |
|---|---|
| ½ | cup fresh lime juice |
| 1 | teaspoons olive oil or olive oil spray |
| 1 | teaspoon chili powder |
| 1 | teaspoon ground cumin |
| 4 | skinless, boneless chicken breast halves (4 ounces each) |
| 2 | medium red bell peppers, cut into wide strips (about 2 cups) |
| 2 | cups cooked pasta |
| 1 | large red onion, cut into wedges |
| 8 | cups mixed salad greens |
| 2 | medium tomatoes, chopped (about 2 cups) |
| ½ | cup chopped green onion |
| ½ | cup chopped carrots several broccoli florets |
| 1 | cup mild or medium salsa |

## Preparation

- Combine lime juice, oil, and spices in shallow glass dish and mix well. Set aside ½ the mixture. Add chicken to dish; turn to coat. Cover dish with plastic wrap and refrigerate 30 minutes.
- Preheat broiler. Drain the chicken and discard marinade. Place on broiler pan and broil three inches from heat, basting with the reserved marinade. Cook about 10 minutes, turning once, until no longer pink in center. Place chicken on a plate; cover to keep warm.
- Place bell peppers and red onion on broiler pan. Broil until lightly charred, turning once, about 8 minutes.
- Coat the pasta with the other half of the lime marinade.
- In a large bowl, add broiled vegetables, mixed greens, raw vegetables, and salsa. Mix gently. Transfer to individual salad bowls, and top with chicken cut into strips.

## Hint

Here's a great meal that's complete as is.

## Per Serving

| | | | |
|---|---|---|---|
| Calories | 375 (14% from fat) | Fat | 6g |
| Carbohydrates | 38g | Protein | 40g |

## Includes

1 serving from Column 1, 1 serving from Column 2 & 4 servings from Column 3 veggie list

# Sue's Chicken Cacciatore

Cacciatore, "hunter" in Italian, indicates food (usually chicken) that is prepared "hunter's style," simmered in a well-seasoned tomato sauce.

## Serves 4

## Ingredients

| | |
|---|---|
| 1 | teaspoon olive oil |
| 4 | cloves garlic, minced |
| 1 | 28 ounce can Italian tomatoes (Pastene Kitchen Ready, Chunky Style) |
| 1 | pound boneless, skinless chicken pieces, cut into chunks |
| 1 | large green pepper cut into strips |
| 1 | large red pepper cut into strips |
| 1 | pound sliced mushrooms (I use ½ domestic white, ½ Portabellas) |
| | Salt & fresh ground pepper |
| | Fresh chopped parsley & basil to taste |
| 4 | cups pasta |

## Preparation

- Sauté garlic in olive oil until fragrant. Add tomatoes, bring to simmer.
- Add chicken; cook for 5 minutes, stirring frequently.
- Add peppers, mushrooms, and spices and simmer over low heat, stirring ocassionally until cooked through (approximately 25 minutes). Serve over pasta

## Hint

To complete this meal add two more peppers.

## Per Serving

| | | | |
|---|---|---|---|
| Calories | 411 (17% from fat) | Fat | 5g |
| Carbohydrates | 50g | Protein | 40g |

## Includes

1 food from Column 1, 2 foods from Column 2 and ½ food from Column 3

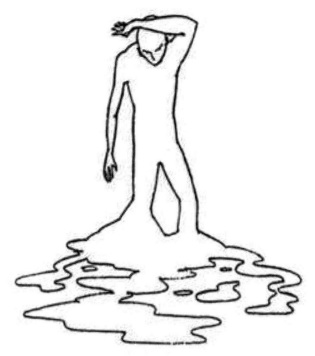

# Chapter 5

# Meatless Meals

# Beans

Beans are an excellent food. They are naturally low-fat and contain lots of dietary fiber. Beans are also high in many vitamins, especially thiamine, riboflavin, niacin, phosphorus, iron , magnesium, zinc, and potassium.

Beans can also be an excellent source of protein when combined with other plant foods to form a complete protein. For persons with high cholesterol, bean dishes should become part of their daily menu planning.

# Tofu

Tofu is made by cooking soybeans with purified water and puréeing the mixture into a creamy soy milk. A precipitant is then added to the milk to separate it into protein-rich curds and liquid. This process concentrates the protein in the soybean to make tofu comparable to meat, fish, poultry, eggs and dairy products in protein quantity.

The distinction from soft tofu to extra firm tofu is determined by water content; the more water the softer the texture. Soft tofu is well suited for creamy dressings, dips, and dessert recipes. Firm tofu is best suited for recipes that call for slicing or dicing and subsequent cooking.

A note of caution. Tofu is a nutritionally valuable food, especially for strict vegetarians. However, regular tofu is high in fat; fifty-two percent of calories are from fat in regular tofu. What's nice about tofu is that only 14 percent of it is saturated; more than half is polyunsaturated. That's easier on your heart than meat, but too much fat in your diet translates to added fat on your body. So, it's important to buy low fat tofu for the following recipes.

# Black Bean Salad

It's so easy to prepare this high protein, healthy bean salad. Canned beans marinated in a tangy citrus vinaigrette give this simple dish a burst of flavor.

## Servings 5

## Ingredients

| | |
|---|---|
| 2 | cans (16 ounces each) black beans, drained |
| 2 | sweet red or green peppers, halved, seeded and diced |
| 5 | green onions, sliced |
| 1 | small red onion, sliced |
| | Juice of 2 lemons |
| | Juice of 2 limes |
| ½ | cup rice wine vinegar or cider vinegar |
| 4 | cloves garlic, finely chopped |
| 1 | tablespoon olive oil |
| | Few drops liquid red pepper seasoning |
| | Salt and freshly ground pepper, to taste |

## Preparation

- In a medium-size bowl combine the black beans, red (or green) pepper, green onion, red onion, lemon and lime juices, rice wine vinegar (or cider vinegar), garlic, oil, liquid red pepper seasoning,
- Cover the bowl and refrigerate the salad. Adjust the seasonings once more before serving, if necessary.

## Hint

To complete this meal garnish with roasted peppers and drink a glass of milk.

## Per Serving

| | | | |
|---|---|---|---|
| Calories | 216 (12.5% from fat) | Fat | 3g |
| Carbohydrates | 36g | Protein | 12g |

## Includes

1 food from Column 1 and ½ food from Column 2

# Tuna & White Bean Salad

Marinating the tuna with low-fat, high fiber white beans allows the flavors of this tasty and healthy salad to develop fully.

## Serves 6

## Ingredients

| | |
|---|---|
| 8 | ounces small dried white beans (pea beans), soaked |
| 1½ | teaspoons salt |
| 1 | jar (2 ounces) sliced pimiento, drained |
| 1 | small red onion, quartered and thinly sliced |
| 1 | can (7 ounces) water-packed tuna, drained and coarsely flaked |
| ¼-⅛ | cup red wine vinegar |
| 2 | tablespoons lemon juice (1 lemon) |
| ½ | teaspoon finely chopped garlic |
| 1 | tablespoon olive oil |
| ¼ | teaspoon freshly ground pepper |
| 2 | tablespoons finely chopped parsley |

Lettuce leaves

Lemon wedges, for garnish (optional)

## Preparation

- Drain white beans; place in medium-size saucepan. Add cold water to saucepan to cover the beans by 2 inches. Bring the water to boil over medium heat. Lower heat. Cover saucepan and simmer beans for 1 hour. Add 1 teaspoon of salt. Cover and simmer for 30 minutes more or until beans are tender but still hold their shape. Drain the beans and place them in a bowl.
- Gently stir the pimiento, onion and tuna into the beans.
- Combine ¼ cup of the vinegar, the lemon juice, garlic, oil, pepper and remaining ½ teaspoon of salt in a small bowl. Stir in parsley. Pour dressing over bean mixture; toss gently to mix all ingredients. Taste and add remaining vinegar, if necessary. Cover bowl; refrigerate salad at least 2 hours, or overnight, to blend the flavors.
- Serve salad on lettuce leaves. Garnish it with lemon wedges. Hint: Serve this salad with a roll and garnish it with raw carrots and broccoli or peppers for a complete meal.

## Per Serving

| | | | |
|---|---|---|---|
| Calories | 280 (12% from fat) | Fat | 4g |
| Carbohydrates | 19g | Protein | 17g |

## Includes

½ food from Column 1and 1 food from Column 2

# Kidney Bean Salad

This salad recipe is low-calorie, low-sodium, and low-cholesterol. For those times when you don't feel like cooking, substituting 2 cups of rinsed and drained canned beans for the dried ones makes a perfect no-cook meal.

## Serves 4

## Ingredients

| | |
|---|---|
| 1 | cup dried kidney beans, soaked overnight |
| 5 | tablespoons lemon juice |
| | Salt and freshly ground pepper, to taste |
| 1 | tablespoon olive oil |
| | Lettuce leaves |
| 1 | sweet green pepper, cored, seeded, and chopped, for garnish |
| ½ | cup chopped green onion, for garnish |
| 3 | tablespoons chopped parsley, for garnish |

## Preparation

- Drain the kidney beans, place them in a saucepan and cover them with fresh water. Bring the water to boil over medium heat. Lower the heat; simmer beans for 1 hour or until they are tender but still whole. Drain the beans.
- Whisk together lemon juice, salt, and pepper in a small bowl. Whisk in the oil until it is blended. Toss the beans with the dressing.
- Spoon the kidney beans into a salad bowl lined with the lettuce leaves. Garnish with the green pepper, green onion and parsley.

## Hint

To complete this meal add more peppers for garnish and serve with a roll and a glass of milk.

## Per Serving

| | | | |
|---|---|---|---|
| Calories | 199 (18% from fat) | Fat | 4g |
| Carbohydrates | 28g | Protein | 11g |

## Includes

½ food from Column 1 & ½ food from Column 2

# Tofu Stuffed Peppers

These delicious stuffed peppers can be prepared and cooked in one hour.

## Serves 4

## Ingredients

| | |
|---|---|
| 4 | small to medium green peppers |
| 4 | sun-dried tomatoes |
| 6 | ounces firm light tofu, drained |
| ½ | cup chopped onion |
| 4 | cloves garlic, chopped |
| 1 | teaspoon crushed dried oregano |
| 1 | teaspoon crushed dried basil |
| 2 | cups cooked brown rice |
| ¼ | cup raisins |
| 1 | cup +¼ cup no salt tomato sauce |
| 1 | tablespoon + 2 teaspoons honey |

pinch cayenne pepper (optional)

## Preparation

- Preheat oven to 350°F.
- Cut tops from peppers, remove seeds and tough inner ribs; steam 4 minutes to soften slightly. Remove peppers from steamer and invert to drain. Place tomatoes in boiling water in steamer base and blanch 2 minutes. Drain and chop.
- Crumble tofu and combine in a skillet with onion and garlic. Saute over medium high heat until tofu is dry. Remove from heat an add sun-dried tomatoes, oregano, basil, brown, rice, raisins, 1 cup tomato sauce and 1 tablespoon honey. Mix well.
- Fill peppers with tofu-rice mixture, stand upright in a baking pan. Mix remaining ¼ cup tomato sauce with remaining 2 teaspoons honey and a pinch of cayenne. Spoon sauce on top of each pepper.
- Pour hot water around peppers to a depth of about 1 inch; bake in a 350°F. oven for 40 minutes, or until peppers are tender and sauce on top is thick.

## Hint

Simply drink a glass of milk to complete this wonderful meal.

## Per Serving

| | | | | |
|---|---|---|---|---|
| Calories | 266 (6% from fat) | | Fat | 2g |
| Carbohydrates | 52g | | Protein | 10g |

## Includes

1 food from Column 1 , ½ food from Column 2 and 1 food from Column 3

# Tofu Mushroom Stuffed Baked Potatoes

## Serves 4

## Ingredients

| | |
|---|---|
| 4 | medium to large baking potatoes |
| 1⅓ | cups chopped onion |
| 1⅓ | cups chopped mushrooms |
| ½ | teaspoon sage |
| | dash white pepper (optional) |
| 8 | ounces firm light tofu, drained and mashed (1½ cups) |
| 3 | tablespoons finely chopped parsley |
| 1 | tablespoon prepared mustard, spicy or dijon |
| ½ | teaspoon honey |
| | paprika for garnish |

## Preparation

- ☐ Bake potatoes in preheated 425°F. oven for 40-60 minutes. In the meantime, you can begin to prepare filling.
- ☐ Combine onion, mushrooms and sage in skillet. Cover and saute 5 minutes over medium heat, until mushrooms become tender and release their juices. Season with white pepper.
- ☐ Cut baked potatoes in half lengthwise and scoop out insides, leaving a shell that is about ¼ inch thick.
- ☐ Combine scooped out potato with tofu, parsley, mustard and honey. Mash together making the mixture as smooth as possible. Stir in mushroom-onion mixture.
- ☐ Fill potato skins with tofu-potato mixture, mounding the filling above the shell. Sprinkle potatoes generously with paprika. Place on baking sheet and bake at 375°F. for 20 minutes.

## Hint

Serve with your favorite veggies from Column 3, and you'll complete this meal.

## Per Serving

| | | | | |
|---|---|---|---|---|
| Calories | 254 (4% from fat) | | Fat | 1g |
| Carbohydrates | 45g | | Protein | 16g |

## Includes

1 food from Column 1 and 1 food from Column 2

# Southwestern Frittata

Prepare and cook this dish in just over half an hour.

## Serves 2

## Ingredients

| | |
|---|---|
| 2-4 | tablespoons fat-free chicken broth |
| 1 | cup thin skinned boiling potatoes, diced |
| ½ | cup chopped onion |
| $\frac{1}{3}$ | cup chopped green pepper |
| ½ | teaspoon +½ teaspoon chili powder |
| 5 | ounces firm light tofu, drained |
| 5 | egg whites |
| 1 | teaspoon honey |
| | pinch cayenne pepper |
| ½ | teaspoon cumin |
| 6 | tablespoon drained salsa |
| | paprika for garnish |

## Preparation

- Steam or boil diced potatoes for 15 minutes or until almost soft.
- In 10-inch nonstick frying pan, sauté potato, onion, and green pepper in chicken broth for 10 minutes or until all vegetables are soft. Stir in ½ teaspoon chili powder.
- Purée tofu with egg whites and honey in blender or food processor. Mix in remaining ½ teaspoon chili powder, cayenne and cumin. Spread vegetables in skillet evenly; pour tofu mixture uniformly over vegetables, cover and cook over low heat about 10 minutes. Add 6 tablespoons drained salsa to center; cook additional 5 minutes or until firm and puffed.
- Garnish with paprika; cut into wedges and serve immediately.

## Try This

Serve frittata with no-salt ketchup or additional salsa.

## Hint

Try serving pita bread and roasted peppers with this meal; it makes a great change and completes the meal.

## Per Serving

| | | | |
|---|---|---|---|
| Calories | 126 (8% from fat) | Fat | 1.5g |
| Carbohydrates | 21g | Protein | 20g |

## Includes

½ food from Column 1and 1 food from Column 2

# Sue's Pasta with Roasted Pepper Sauce

Roasting peppers takes a little bit of time, but it is well worth it for the flavor! Use roasted peppers on sandwiches too!

## Serves 4

## Ingredients

| | |
|---|---|
| 1 | teaspoon olive oil |
| 2 | cups onion, chopped |
| 4 | cloves garlic, minced |
| ½ | teaspoon fennel seeds, crushed |
| 2 | 28 ounce cans No-Salt Added whole tomatoes undrained and chopped |
| 1 | pound red peppers, roasted and peeled (see directions) |
| 1 | pound green peppers, roasted and peeled (see directions) |
| 1 | pound yellow peppers, roasted and peeled (see directions) |
| ½ | teaspoon salt and fresh ground pepper to taste |
| ½ | bunch thinly sliced fresh basil |
| 4 | cups cooked pasta |

## Preparations

- Sauté onion, fennel seeds, and garlic in olive oil until tender, about 5 minutes, stirring occasionally.
- Add tomatoes, bring to simmer.
- Add pepper strips, salt, and pepper, and half of the basil. Simmer on low heat, stirring occasionally, about 45 minutes.
- Serve over pasta, sprinkle with remaining basil and fresh grated parmesan cheese.

## For Roasting Peppers

- Cut peppers in half lengthwise; discard seeds and membranes. Place peppers, skin side up on a foil lined baking sheet, flatten with palm of hand.
- Broil (close to heat) until blackened and charred (about 10 minutes).
- Place in zip-lock heavy-duty plastic bag, seal and let stand 15 minutes or so. Remove from bag, peel and discard skins.

## Hint:

Drink a glass of milk to complete this meal.

## Per Serving

| | | | |
|---|---|---|---|
| Calories | 271 (16% from fat) | Fat | 3g |
| Carbohydrates | 51g | Protein | 10g |

## Includes

1 food from Column 1, ½ food from Column 2 and 1 food from Column 3

# Janine's No-Fat Chili Rice & Bean Casserole

Just mix and microwave this dish. It makes a great, quick lunch or dinner and it's a perfect lunch to take to work.

## Serves 4

## Ingredients

| | |
|---|---|
| 2 | cups cooked rice |
| 1½ | cups no-fat cottage cheese |
| 1 | cup red beans |
| 1 | cup black beans |
| ½ | cup Healthy Choice spaghetti sauce |
| 1 | pound bag cooked spinach |
| 1 | tablespoon chile powder |

## Preparation

- Mix all ingredients and microwave until hot.
- Portion out into approximately 1½ cup servings.

## Hint

To make a complete meal just add a salad!

## Per Serving

| | | | |
|---|---|---|---|
| Calories | 240 (0% from fat) | Fat | 0g |
| Carbohydrates | 40g | Protein | 20g |

## Includes

1 food from Column 1, 1 food from Column 2 and ½ food from Column 3

# Janine's Low-Fat Spinach Lasagna

A great-tasting, meatless, low-fat alternative to traditional lasagna!

## Serves 4

## Ingredients

| | |
|---|---|
| 1 | pound fresh cooked spinach |
| 16 | ounce can whole tomatoes |
| ½ | cup Healthy Choice Non-Fat Cheddar |
| ½ | cup Healthy Choice Non-Fat Mozzarella |
| ½ | teaspoon + ½ teaspoon chili powder |
| 1 | cup non-fat cottage cheese |
| 2 | tablespoons grated cheese |
| 2 | cups tomato purée |
| 8 | ounces lasagna noodles |
| 1 | tablespoon Italian seasoning |
| | salt and pepper |

## Preparation

- Boil pasta for 5 minutes.
- Combine purée, salt, pepper (to taste), Italian seasoning, and juice from the canned tomatoes. Mix in cheeses (except grated cheese).
- Place enough sauce mixture on the bottom of a lasagna pan to cover.
- Add a row of lasagna noodles, then a layer of spinach, then a layer of sauce.
- Next add another layer of noodles and then the whole tomatoes. Add cheeses and the remainder of the sauce and sprinkle with grated cheese.
- Bake 45 minutes to 1 hour at 350°F. Be sure to let lasagna set for 15 minutes to thicken before serving.

## Hint

Add a nice salad to complete this meal.

## Per Serving

| | | | | |
|---|---|---|---|---|
| Calories | 322 (6% from fat) | | Fat | 2g |
| Carbohydrates | 51g | | Protein | 25g |

## Includes

1 food from Column 1, 1 food from Column 2 and ½ food from Column 3

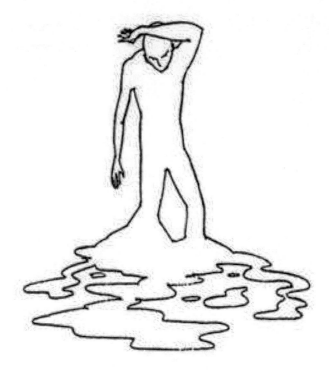

# Chapter 6
# Perfect Endings

# About Baking

Fat has traditionally been used in baked goods like cakes and cookies to add moistness and tenderness. Fat can be totally eliminated or dramatically reduced by using healthier alternatives.

Fruit fat substitutes: Fruit purees, applesauce, and fruit juices can replace all of the fat in cakes, muffins, quick breads, scones, and brownies. Fruit substitutes can replace at least half of the fat in cookies.

Dairy fat substitutes: Nonfat yogurt and buttermilk can replace all of the fat in cakes, muffins, quick breads, scones, biscuits, and brownies, and at least half of the fat in cookies.

Sweet fat substitutes: Liquid sweeteners like honey, molasses, jam, corn syrup, and chocolate syrup can replace all of the fat in cakes, muffins, quick breads, scones, biscuits, brownies, cookies, crumb toppings, and sweet crumb crusts.

Prunes: Easy to make prune butter and prune puree can replace all of the fat in cakes, muffins, quick breads, scones, brownies, cookies, and sweet crumb crusts. (See banana creme pie recipe.)

Squash and sweet potato: Mashe pumpkin, other mashed squashes, and sweet potatoes can replace all of the fat in cakes, quick breads, muffins, biscuits, scones, and brownies, and at least half of the fat in cookies.

Reduced-fat margarine and light butter: Reduced-fat margarine and light butter can cut the fat in biscuits, scones, cakes, muffins, quick breads, cookies, brownies, pie crusts, and crumb toppings by more than half.

In many baked products protein can be increased by adding powdered milk to any milk already in the recipe; powdered milk can also be added to flour.

# Maximizing Moistness

The most common complaint about fat free baking is that the baked goods are too dry. Here are some important hints to keep in mind when creating fat free treats:

Avoid overbaking. Fat free treats bake more quickly than those made with fat. Baked at too high a temperature or left in the oven too long will produce dryness.

Use the toothpick test. The best way to check fat free baked products is to insert a toothpick in the center of the product. As soon as the toothpick comes out clean, the product should be removed from the oven. Remove fat free brownies from the oven as soon as the edges are firm and the center is almost set.

Keep baked goods moist and fresh. Fat free baked goods have a high moisture content and no preservatives. To keep these products at their freshest, place them in an airtight container and arrange them in single layers separated by sheets of waxed paper. Leftovers should be refrigerated for maximum freshness.

# Carrot Cake

If you love carrot cake, you'll love this almost fat free version. No guilt when eating this cake!

## 16 Servings

## Ingredients

2½    cups unbleachedflour
1¼    cups brown sugar
2     teaspoons baking soda
2     teaspoons ground cinnamon
¾     cup plus 2 tablespoons apple juice
4     egg whites
2     teaspoons vanilla extract
3     cups grated carrots (about 6 medium)
⅓     cup dark raisins

## Cream Cheese Icing

8     ounces nonfat cream cheese
1     cup nonfat ricotta cheese
½     cup confectioners' sugar
1     teaspoon vanilla extract

## Preparation

☐   Combine the flour, brown sugar, baking soda, and cinnamon, and stir to mix well. Add the juice, egg whites, and vanilla extract, and stir well. Stir in the carrots and the raisins.

☐   Coat a 9 x 13 inch pan with nonstick cooking spray. Spread the batter evenly in the pan and bake at 325°F for 40 to 50 minutes, or just until a wooden toothpick inserted in the center comes out clean. Cool to room temperature.

☐   To make the icing, place the cream cheese and ricotta in a food processor, and process until smooth. Add the confectioners' sugar and vanilla extract, and process to mix well. Spread the icing over the cooled cake. Cut into squares and serve immediately or refirgerate.

## Per Slice

| | | |
|---|---|---|
| Calories | 205 (< 1% from fat) | Fat 0.3g |
| Carbohydrates | 42g | Protein 8g |

## Includes

1 food from Column 1, ½ food from Column 2 and ¼ food from Column 3

# Real Fudge Brownies

These brownies are "almost" as good as the real thing. They satisfy any sweet tooth.

## 16 Servings

## Ingredients

| | |
|---|---|
| ¾ | cup unbleached flour |
| ¼ | cup plus 2 tablespoons cocoa powder |
| 1 | cup sugar |
| ¹/₃ | cup unsweetened applesauce |
| 3 | egg whites |
| ¼ | cup chopped walnuts (optional) |
| ¼ | teaspoon salt (optional) |
| 1 | teaspoon vanilla extract |

## Preparation

- Combine the flour, cocoa, sugar, and stir to mix well. Stir in the applesauce, egg whites, and vanilla extract (fold in nuts if desired).
- Coat an 8 inch pan with nonstick cooking spray. Spread the batter evenly in the pan and bake at 325°F for 23 to 25 minutes, or just until the edges are firm and the center is almost set.
- Cool to room temperature, cut into squares and serve.

## Per Brownie

| | | | |
|---|---|---|---|
| Calories | 80 (< 1% from fat) | Fat | 0.4g |
| Carbohydrates | 18g | Protein | 1.6g |

## Includes

½ food from Column 1

# Oatmeal Cookies

Great cookies even the "kids" will love (even those big kids).

## 50 Cookies

## Ingredients

| | |
|---|---|
| 3 | cups quick cooking oats |
| 1 | cup whole wheat flour |
| 1 | teaspoon baking soda |
| ¼ | teaspoon ground nutmeg |
| 1 | cup unsweetened apple sauce |
| 1 | cup sugar |
| 1 | teaspoon vanilla extract |
| ²/₃ | cup dark raisins |

## Preparation

- Combine the oats, flour, baking soda, and nutmeg, and stir to mix well. Add the applesauce, sugar, vanilla extract, and stir to mix well. Stir in the raisins.
- Coat cookie sheets with nonstick cooking spray. Roll the dough into one inch balls and place 1 ½ inches apart on the cookie sheets. If the dough is sticky place in the freezer for a few minutes. Flatten the cookies to ¼ inch thickness using the bottom of a glass dipped in sugar.
- Bake at 275°F for 22 minutes, or until lightly browned.
- Transfer cookies to wire rack, and cool to room temperature.

## Per Cookie

| | | | |
|---|---|---|---|
| Calories | 49 (< 1% from fat) | Fat | 0.3g |
| Carbohydrates | 11g | Protein | 1.2g |

## Includes

½ food from Column 1

# Raspberry Scones

If you are a "scone" lover, you'll definitely want to add this one to your library.

## 12 scones

## Ingredients

| | |
|---|---|
| 1 | cup quick cooking oats |
| 1½ | cups unbleached flour |
| 2 | tablespoons sugar |
| 2 | teaspoons baking powder |
| ½ | teaspoon baking soda |
| 1 | egg white |
| ¾ | cup plus 2 tablespoons lemon or vanilla nonfat yogurt |
| ½ | cup chopped fresh or frozen raspberries |

skim milk or 1 beaten egg white

## Preparation

- Combine the oats, flour, sugar, baking powder, baking soda, and stir to mix well. Stir in the egg white and just enough of the yogurt to form a stiff dough. Gently stir in the rasberries.
- Form the dough into a ball, and turn onto a lightly floured surface. With floured hands, pat the dough into a 7 inch circle. Coat a baking sheet with nonstick cooking spray. Place the dough on the sheet, and use a sharp floured knife to cut it into 12 wedges. Pull the wedges out slightly to leave 1/2 inch space between them. Brush the tops lightly with skim milk or beaten egg white.
- Bake at 375°F for 20 minutes, or until lightly browned.
- Transfer to a serving plate, and serve hot with raspberry fruit spread

## Per Scone

| | | | |
|---|---|---|---|
| Calories | 112 (< 1% from fat) | Fat | 0.5g |
| Carbohydrates | 23g | Protein | 3.8g |

## Includes

1 food from Column 1

# Cocoa Bundt Cake

This cake is always a big hit!

## 16 servings

## Ingredients

2¼    cups unbleached flour
¾    cup oat bran
1⅓    cups sugar
4½    teaspoons lecithin granules*
1¼    teaspoons baking soda
1⅔    cups nonfat buttermilk
2    egg whites
1½    teaspoons vanilla extract
¼    cup chocolate syrup
¼    cup cocoa powder

## Glaze:

⅓  cup confectioners' sugar
1  tablespoon cocoa powder
2  teaspoons skim milk
½  teaspoon vanilla extract

## Preparation

- Combine the flour, oat bran, sugar, lecithin, and baking soda, and stir to mix well. Add the buttermilk, egg whites, vanilla extract, and stir to mix well. Remove 1 cup of the batter and mix with the chocolate syrup and cocoa powder.
- Coat bundt pan with nonstick cooking spray. Spread 3/4 of the plain batter evenly in the pan, top with the chocolate mixture, and add the remaining batter.
- Bake at 350°F for 35 to 45 minutes, or until wooden toothpick inserted in the center of the cake comes out clean.
- Cool in pan for 20 minutes. Transfer cake to serving platter. Make glaze by combining ingredients, stirring until smooth. Drizzle glaze over cake. Let sit for at least 15 minutes before slicing and serving.

## Per Slice

| | | | |
|---|---|---|---|
| Calories | 174 (< 1% from fat) | Fat | 1.3g |
| Carbohydrates | 37g | Protein | 4.1g |

## Includes

1 food from Column 1

# Blueberry Streusel Cake

Another award winning low fat cake!

## 9 servings

## Ingredients

| | |
|---|---|
| ²/₃ | cup skim milk |
| 2 | tablespoons lemon juice |
| 1½ | cups unbleached flour |
| ½ | cup oat flour |
| ½ | cup sugar |
| 4 | teaspoons baking powder |
| 1 | teaspoon dried grated lemon rind, or 1 tablespoon fresh |
| 1 | egg white |
| 1½ | cups fresh or frozen blueberries |

## Glaze:

| | |
|---|---|
| ¼ | cup quick cooking oats |
| 1 | tablespoon wheat germ |
| ⅛ | teaspoon ground nutmeg |
| 2 | teaspoons honey |

## Preparation

- To make the topping, combine the oats, wheat germ, and nutmeg. Stir in the honey until the mixture is moist and crumbly. Set aside.
- Combine the milk and lemon juice, and set aside for 2 minutes. Combine the flours, sugar, baking powder, lemon rind, and stir to mix well. Stir in the lemon juice mixture and the egg white. Fold in the blueberries.
- Coat an 8 inch pan with nonstick cooking spray. Spread the batter evenly in the pan, and sprinkle with the topping.
- Bake at 350°F for 35 to 45 minutes, or until wooden toothpick inserted in the center of the cake comes out clean.
- Cool for 20 minutes. Cut into squares and serve warm or at room temperature.

## Per Slice

| | | | |
|---|---|---|---|
| Calories | 184 (< 1% from fat) | Fat | .9g |
| Carbohydrates | 39g | Protein | 5g |

## Includes

1 food from Column 1

# Black Forest Cake

Wow!  Black Forest Cake with less than 1 gram of fat per serving!

## 10 servings

## Ingredients

| | |
|---|---|
| 1 | cup unbleached flour |
| ½ | cup oat bran |
| ¾ | cup sugar |
| ¼ | cup cocoa powder |
| 1 | teaspoon baking soda |
| 1 | teaspoon vanilla extract |
| ¼ | cup chocolate syrup |
| 1½ | teaspoons white vinegar |
| 1 | cup water |

## Filling

| | |
|---|---|
| 1 | can (20oz) lt cherry pie filling |

## Merinque Topping

| | |
|---|---|
| 2 | egg whites (room temp) |
| ⅛ | teaspoon cream of tartar |
| 5 | tablespoons sugar |
| 1 | teaspoon vanilla extract |

## Preparation

- Combine the flours, sugar, cocoa, baking soda, and stir to mix well. In a separate bowl, combine the vanilla extract, chocolate syrup, vinegar, and water.  Add the chocolate mixture to the flour mixture and stir to mix well.
- Coat a 10 inch flan pan with nonstick cooking spray.  Spread the batter evenly in the pan.
- Bake at 350°F for 15 to 20 minutes, or until wooden toothpick inserted in the center of the cake comes out clean.
- Cool to room temperature.  Invert onto a baking sheet.  Fill the depression in the top of the cake with the cherry pie filling.
- Make meringue topping by whipping the egg whites and cream of tartar with an electric mixer until soft peaks form.  Still beating, slowly add the sugar and vanilla extract.  Continue to beat until stiff peaks form.
- Spoon the meringue in a ring around the outer edge of the cherry filling.  Place the cake in a 400°F oven for 3 to 5 minutes, or until the meringue is lightly browned.  Cool the cake to room temperature. Slice and serve immediately, or refrigerate to prevent the merinque from separating.

## Per Slice

| | | | |
|---|---|---|---|
| Calories | 219(< 1% from fat) | Fat | .9g |
| Carbohydrates | 49g | Protein | 3.4g |

## Includes

1 food from Column 1

# Peach Pie

You can use any favorite fruit filling for this low fat alternative.

## 8 servings

## Ingredients

**Crunchy Crust**
5   ounces (2½ cups) oat flakes ready to eat cereal
3   tablespoons fruit spread or jam (any flavor)

**Filling**
3   cups sliced fresh peaches (4 medium)
1   cup fresh blueberries

**Glaze**
⅓  cup sugar
1½ cups peach nectar
3   tablespoons cornstarch

## Preparation

- Crust: place the cereal in the bowl of a food processsor or in a blender. Process into fine crumbs. Measure the crumbs. There should be 1¼ cups. Return the crumbs to the food processor, and add the fruit spread. Process until moist and crumbly.
- Coat a 9 inch pie pan with nonstick cooking spray. Using the back of a spoon, press the crumbs against the sides and bottom of the pan, forming an even crust. Periodically dip the spoon in sugar, to prevent sticking. Bake pie shell at 350°F for 10 to 12 minutes, or until edges feel firm and dry. Cool crust to room temperature.
- Make glaze by combining the sugar and cornstarch in a medium sized saucepan. Slowly stir in the nectar. Place over medium heat and bring to a boil, stirring constantly. Reduce the heat to low, and cook for another minute. Remove the saucepan from the heat, and set aside for 15 minutes.
- Stir the glaze, and spoon a thin layer over the bottom of the pie crust. Arrange half of the peachers in a circular pattern over the bottom of the crust. Top with blueberries, and spoon half of the remaining glaze over the berries. Arrange the rest of the peachers over the glaze, and top with the remaining glaze.
- Chill for several hours. Cut into wedges and serve cold.

## Per Slice

| | | | |
|---|---|---|---|
| Calories | 193(< 1% from fat) | Fat | .3g |
| Carbohydrates | 45g | Protein | 2.7g |

## Includes

1 food from Column 1

# Strawberry Cheesecake

One of Dr. Jane's favorites!

## 10 servings

## Ingredients

| | |
|---|---|
| ²/₃ | cup low sugar strawberry preserves |
| 2 | containers (15 ounces each) nonfat ricotta cheese |
| ½ | cup nonfat sour cream or plain nonfat yogurt |
| 6 | egg whites |
| ²/₃ | cup sugar |
| ¼ | cup unbleached flour |
| 2 | teaspoons vanilla extract |

## Crunchy Crust

| | |
|---|---|
| 5 | ounces (2½ cups) oat flakes ready to eat cereal |
| 3 | tablespoons fruit spread or jam (any flavor) |

## Preparation

☐ Coat a 9 inch springform pan with nonstick cooking spray. Prepare crust: place the cereal in the bowl of a food processsor or in a blender. Process into fine crumbs. Measure the crumbs. There should be 1¼ cups. Return the crumbs to the food processor, and add the fruit spread. Process until moist and crumbly. Using the back of a spoon, press the crumbs against the sides (½ inch up) and bottom of the pan, forming an even crust. Periodically dip the spoon in sugar, to prevent sticking. Bake pie shell at 350°F for 8 minutes, or until edges feel firm and dry. Cool crust to room temperature.

☐ Place jam in a microwave, uncovered at 50 percent power for 2 minutes or until runny. Set aside.

☐ Place the ricotta, sour cream or yogurt, egg whites in food processor and process until smooth. Add sugar, flour, vanilla extract, and process until smooth. Spread ½ of the cheese filling evenly over the crust. Spoon half of the heated jam randomly over the filling. Top with remaining filling. Spoon rest of jam randomly over top. Draw a knife through the batter to produce a marbled effect.

☐ Bake at 350 for 60 to 70 minutes, or until center is set. Turn oven off and allow cake to cool in the oven with door ajar for 30 minutes. Chill for at least 8 hours. Remove the collar of the pan just before slicing and serving.

## Per Slice

| | | | |
|---|---|---|---|
| Calories | 239(< 1% from fat) | Fat | 1.0g |
| Carbohydrates | 43g | Protein | 15g |

## Includes

1 food from Column 1 and 1 food from Column 2

LaVergne, TN USA
01 June 2010

184554LV00004B/2/P